Foreword

I sit down to write this e-book; and as I sit, I realize it will be so easy to write, there will be no writer's block, in fact I expect to have the whole book written in maybe just 4 days!

Why? Because I am so excited to tell you what I have found out over the last year with my so-called (if you listen to doctors) "dangerous experiment", that I can't wait to get it all down!

A Second Foreword

Yes. I did in fact write the first draft of this book in about 4 days. I started with some notes on my experiment which seemed more like material taken from a diary than fodder for a book. I tried to mold these lab notes and diary entries into a book mixed with other information like evolutionary theory and various interesting facts and insights. And I kept updating the book with newer and sometimes more correct information than had been in it before. So the book reads more like a diary of a journey into the unknown rather than a hyper-edited reference guide. While some may find this a difficult style of writing to read, I believe it offers the reader a better appreciation of what a self-experiment with high dose Vitamin D3 will be like.

1.
The Whole Book in a Nut Shell

Let me spill some of the really interesting tidbits first right now before we get started, just to whet your appetite. After all my experimentation and researching and thinking about Vitamin D3, I have stumbled upon a very simple theory about D3 that is elegant in its simplicity.

This simple theory can be created from combining just a few simple facts and a little common sense. This simple theory just might be able to explain the cause of, or how to prevent most of the diseases and health problems that humans face (with the exception of aging-related diseases and syndromes from genetic mutations). Everything else it seems, I have found, might just be preventable or curable by careful, occasional super-high dose Vitamin D3 therapy.

Okay, I will now describe the major relevant facts and ideas regarding what I call The Human Hibernation Syndrome which is caused by your body not getting enough sun and thus acting as if it is preparing for winter.

Fact 1:

Vitamin D3 is not a vitamin! It is actually a seco-steroid hormone that affects almost all the cells in your body by altering the expression of your genes. Vitamin D3 receptors are found in all the cells of your body.

Fact 2:

Vitamin D3 is the active hormone form of Vitamin D and people used to generally get most of their Vitamin D3 from exposing their skin to the sun. The sun activates an inactive form of Vitamin D which is actually very similar to and made from cholesterol, and turns it into the functioning hormone. (There are a few other minor steps in the kidneys and liver but we can ignore them for our purposes). Vitamin D2 and D1 are much less active plant-derived forms of the hormone that you can get from your diet if you eat amongst other things UV irradiated mushrooms. D1 and D2 are considered inferior synthetic, weak, versions of the animal hormone D3. (There are a large number of hormones that are made from chole**stero**l as the starting point. That's why they call them **stero**ids, and it includes hormones such as, Vitamin D3, testo**stero**ne, estrogen, DHEA, proge**stero**ne, cortisol, etc. They are all very similar looking except for a few tiny tweaks here and there).

Fact 3:

People generally make a lot more Vitamin D3 with their skin in the summer sunny months than in the dark winter months. Although D3 can be acquired from the diet and diet now might be the primary source of D3 for many, most people used to get the majority of their D3 from sun exposure.

Fact 4:

Vitamin D3 deficiency is associated with a huge number of diseases and disorders. Let us focus just on obesity, depression, arthritis, and susceptibility to the common cold for now.

Now here is the logic: In the spring and summer your body is exposed to lots of sun, and thus your Vitamin D3 levels are high and rising. Your body, from an evolutionary perspective believes that food is abundant, days are long, and everything is good. So the sunshine hormone D3 tells your body it's okay to burn a lot of energy and get things done, because food and vitamin resources will be available. Thus from D3 you get lots of energy; it keeps you active; keeps your hunger under control, and keeps you healthy (as will be described shortly).

When winter arrives in the northern latitudes northern residents have a dramatic reduction in the production of D3- the sunshine hormone signal. From an evolutionary perspective your body now expects a good chance of famine conditions that often occur around winter when resources are scarce. (Just ask the Donner party about winter famine! The pioneers began to starve to death in 1846 on a Nevada mountain trail in a blizzard. They were reduced to cannibalism to survive, leaving just 48 survivors out of 87 in the original party!)

Now, if you happened to be a northern bear, declining and low D3 would be one of the signals to tell you to begin to get ready to hibernate. In fact in black bears Vitamin D3 levels are at about 23 nmol/L in the summer (around 10 ng/mL which is the scale we usually use) and decline to 8 nmol/L (or 3 ng/mL) during hibernation with the drop in D3 being offset by a large increase in an inactive form of Vitamin D, which in the bear's case is a pseudo-Vitamin D2. A bear

preparing for hibernation will begin to eat as much as possible to put on as much weight as it can to get ready to wait out the winter. Female bears often increase their weight from their lowest summer weight to hibernation weight by 70%. Many other mammals hibernate including raccoons, skunks, woodchucks, chipmunks, hamsters, hedgehogs, and bats. Most reptiles and amphibians hibernate as well as crocodiles and alligators that go for months without eating when it is cold and darker. Apparently, hibernation is a response that might have evolved in all animals or their evolutionary ancestors from time to time. With this in mind, it is highly likely that we humans have some sort of ancient but semi-suppressed hibernation mechanisms locked up in our DNA.

2.
Hibernation

If you doubt that humans might have evolved from a hibernating ancestor, you would also likely doubt that dogs evolved from a hibernating canine-right? Well take a look at the Raccoon Dog-considered a primitive/ancient version of the canine and this dog still exists today:

An excerpt from the Wikipedia entry for "Raccoon Dog":

> Raccoon dogs are the only canids known to hibernate in winter. In early winter, they increase their subcutaneous fat by 18–23% and their internal fat by 3–5%. Animals failing to reach these fat levels usually do not survive the winter period. During their winter sleep, their metabolism decreases by 25%. In areas such as Ussuriland and their introduced range, raccoon dogs only hibernate during severe snowstorms. In December, their physical activity decreases once snow depth reaches 15–20 cm, and will not vacate their burrows for more than 150–200 m. Their daily activities increase during February when the females become receptive and when food is more available.[2]

So we must ask is it possible that humans have a hibernation response somewhat similar to other mammals where when we are affected by low levels of D3 (from low levels of sunshine hitting our skin) that we crave carbohydrates, and put on lots of weight, and then we get depressed so that we slow down and don't waste so much precious energy? Can evolution slow us down by allowing us to get sick with the common cold which is usually harmless (and to which we are normally immune in the summer) but keeps us bedridden for a week or so in the winter and thus further saves precious energy? Could evolution also want to slow us down by giving us aches and pains from arthritis to keep us housebound and to keep us from using up potentially scarce energy resources? I think the answer is YES! (Now an alternative idea to aches and pains being used by evolution to slow us down is that evolution just does not repair us completely while hibernating, but rather just enough to get by, to conserve potentially critical resources for other possible future crises- Imagine that your body knows you are about to go through a three month famine and you break your arm, will your body use <u>all</u> its calcium stores to fix your arm, or fix your arm just enough to get by? What if you had a second or third break during the famine months? Would there be any calcium left to fix those breaks if your body used up all your calcium on your first broken bone?-this idea will be developed later).

Fact 5:

Obese people, depressed people, and people with arthritis or general musculoskeletal pains have been found to be overwhelmingly deficient in Vitamin D3!

Fact 6:

Experiments have been performed in prison where 100% of the inmate population every winter would get the common flu. One experiment where they gave everyone, in one cell block only, Vitamin D3 supplements, 100% of the prisoners in Cell Block D3 were protected from getting the common cold!

Fact 7:

Since the early 1980's, when doctors started warning us about too much sun, obesity rates in adults humans and many other diseases (including asthma and autism) have skyrocketed!

Fact 8:

It was in the early 1980's that doctors have been telling us to avoid the sun to prevent skin cancer and to use lots of high-strength sun block anytime one went outside.

3.
The Human Hibernation Syndrome

So the bottom line simple theory developed from these facts is that if you don't get enough Vitamin D3, evolution expects a winter-long famine might come soon and tries to get you to hibernate until the spring and summer sun returns. Thus if you never get back in the sun again after winter you will suffer from a permanent case of what I call the Human Hibernation Syndrome.

The Incomplete Repair Syndrome

A subset theory of this theory which can also explain the many other diseases and conditions caused by low vitamin D3 levels is what I call- the Incomplete Repair Syndrome. This is a syndrome where evolution has designed us to stingily conserve our critical resources and only uses them very sparingly to fix injuries and do common maintenance of the body. This stinginess leads to incomplete repairs and maintenance that will be completed just enough to get by. The body will stay in this mode until it gets the sunshine hormone signal that tells it that resources will now again be abundant, and the body can go ahead and undo the incomplete repairs and maintenance and redo them thoroughly, properly, and completely, using all the resources necessary.

So that's it. If you, like most people, have chronically low Vitamin D3 levels all year and eventually all life long, you will eventually get depressed, obese, sick, and will begin to accumulate injuries that never heal, and maintenance issues that never go away! And since 1980 when doctors started convincing us to stay out of the sun and use strong sun block, a huge portion of the US population has become obese. And a lot of other problems are becoming apparent like an explosive rise in autism, asthma, and even dangerous peanut allergies.

So that's the underlying theory for this whole book in a nut shell. Now let's begin with a little background.

4.
The History of Vitamin D3

Let me give you a several paragraph history about Vitamin D3 that might get you interested in knowing more:

Vitamin D has been known to exist in some manner by mankind supposedly back to antiquity, but it wasn't until around 1650 that the first case of Vitamin D deficiency was described scientifically (called Rickets). And it wasn't until around 1920 that a scientist that experimented with dogs that were raised 100% indoors and completely out of the sun, figured out that if you fed them a little cod liver oil that they would not get Rickets. Rickets, it was found, could also be cured by exposure of the dogs to sunlight. Later it was discovered that the active compound in cod liver oil was none other than Vitamin D3!

What is Rickets? It is a bone disease which ran rampant amongst the European and US city populations back in the 1800's and early 1900's when everyone was working indoors in factories and not getting enough sun. Kids with Rickets ended up with stunted growth, bowed legs, and soft and weak bones while women would get deformations in their pelvises so severe that they had to get C-sections to give birth. When adults got Rickets they gave it a different name, osteomalacia, which roughly means "bone badness".

Because something in cod liver oil cured a deficiency they called that substance "Vitamin D" because they had only discovered Vitamins A, B and C before this new discovery. Little did they know that it was not a vitamin at all, but actually a vital steroid hormone (technically a seco-steroid) that seems to be essential to most life forms for good health. Vitamin D3 was found in cod liver oil, (the cod make it too) but it can also be created by our own bodies when we sit in the sun and the sun hits our unprotected skin. The same goes for dogs, cats, rats and most other forms of life. Somehow the sun gets past their fur and causes them to make Vitamin D3 too. (Actually later I learned that hairy mammals and birds secrete an oily substance onto their fur or feathers which is very similar to Vitamin D2, the sun then hits it and converts it into D3, and these animals then get their necessary D3 when they groom themselves and lick up the D3 which was converted by the sun from the D2-like substance). Thus Vitamin D3 will be good for your dogs and cats and other pets-just like it is for us! I can just imagine how Vitamin D3 (plus Vitamin K2-more on K2 later) should be able to help all those large breed dogs that seem so susceptible to arthritis. D3 supplementation from birth for your pets should also prevent them from becoming fat cats and dogs.

Well this was a major breakthrough! And scientists found that all that was needed to keep one's bones from going soft, or growth being retarded, or one's pelvis from growing deformed was a small dose of about 400 IU a day of Vitamin D (or just a little sunlight on your skin for a few minutes). And until just last year when the "Institute of Medicine" raised the recommended dose of D3 to 800 to 2000 IU a day, 400 IU was the recommended daily allowance of Vitamin D…Only 400 IU a day! – just enough to keep you from dying or suffering debilitating soft bone disease!

And until 2011, that is basically all we have been getting in our Multi Vitamins unless we go out and sunbathe (without sun block).

20 mg's of Vitamin D in the 1920's becomes 1,000,000 IU's in the 1930's

IU is just a standard drug measurement like an inch is to length...it stands for International Units and means nothing more

-later (after the first edition of this book) I learned that supposedly IU's were invented by Big Pharma to confuse the public to prevent them from taking high dose Vitamin D3 instead of Big Pharma's expensive drugs (20 mg's of D3 = 1,000,000 IU's!)- See update #4 at the end of this book-before the reader feedback. This of course assumes some sort of conspiratorial effort on the part of Big Pharma to scare consumers away from taking D3 so they will instead buy Big Pharma's expensive drugs! More on this later.)

Toxicity

Soon after the discovery of Vitamin D, scientists also discovered Vitamin D toxicity. The toxicity occurs because Vitamin D does not flush right through your body like Vitamin C does, but rather it can accumulate in your fatty tissues, and if you get WAY TOO MUCH Vitamin D stored up, you can have some problems. In the worst cases (which are almost unknown) Vitamin D toxicity can promote heart disease, can "attack" the joints, cause kidney damage, give you hypertension, and excess calcification here and there. Scary I bet you say!

By contrast Rickets/Vitamin D deficiency causes loss of calcium from the bones which then enters the blood, which can also mess up your joints through arthritic calcification, and also cause heart disease and an AMAZING amount of other bad things as you soon will see. So it seems like you're damned if you do and damned if you don't! Trust me, however, when you are done reading this e-book you will realize everyone has a level that is "just right" and odds are probably 100 to 1 that your Vitamin D3 levels are on the *way too low* side for optimal health. You, my friend, are almost 99% guaranteed to be Vitamin D3 deficient, if not by today's standards, then definitely by tomorrow's.

Well it turns out that Vitamin D toxicity was and is a *very rare* occurrence and only occurred/s from a normal person ingesting super high amounts of Vitamin D, like in the one million IU's per day range- for months at a time, and when these over-ingesting people stopped the massive doses they were accidentally taking, they basically returned to normal but in some cases had reduced kidney function and increased blood pressure probably due to calcification of the kidneys and arteries (likely from an induced Vitamin K2 deficiency). If this sounds like a risk, you will soon learn that the risks of having too low Vitamin D3 levels are many times worse for you!

Vitamin D toxicity is said to have *never* occurred from too much sun exposure. From one Doctor's website… "The early cases of vitamin D toxicity that formed the basis for safety concerns generally involved impurities in vitamin D production, the use of synthetic vitamin D analogues, accidental use of extremely high doses, or individuals with vitamin D hypersensitivity. For various reasons, vitamin D toxicity became an issue of exaggerated concern, the extent of which is only now becoming evident. Looking back, scientists now realize that vitamin D toxicity is rare and generally occurs from extremely high oral intake, never from sunlight exposure." (From-Nutrition & bone health Vitamin D: An old bone builder takes on new importance. *Dr. Susan E. Brown, PhD)*

I did a little research about vitamin D toxicity and searched all the science journal articles on it since 1967 to present in the Pub Med database and discovered that Vitamin D3 toxicity even at really high amounts almost never occurs, and most of the articles describe super high doses people have taken without any damage. The articles were published because the doctors were dumbfounded! The results they saw contradicted everything they had learned about the evils of Vitamin D in med school. I also discovered there might be a subset of about 5% of the population who are more sensitive to very high Vitamin D doses than the rest of the population.

The Importance of Vitamin K2 (Not K1)

However the new prevailing theory about vitamin D toxicity is that it is caused by the body's depletion of Vitamin K2 because higher doses of Vitamin D cause certain reactions in your body that use up your Vitamin K2. So maybe the 5% are just extra deficient in Vitamin K2 and nothing more. So just a little reminder here, if you decide to embark on a "dangerous" experiment of Super-High Dose Vitamin D3, DEFINITELY make sure you take about two or three Vitamin K2 supplements every day as well. Keep in mind K1 cannot substitute for K2- K1 helps clot your blood while K2 keeps the calcium in your bones and out of your blood and soft tissues. Additionally there are 2 kinds of K2 : MK-4 from animal products, And MK-7 from bacteria. Supposedly the MK-7 is the good stuff, much stronger and lasts longer and there is no toxicity with K2 so take as much as you want! (I will add a caveat to this advice later.)

Wait! Let me emphasize this point one more time since I have been getting emails from people deciding to take high dose D3 without taking vitamin K2. Do not take a lot of D3 unless you also take a lot of vitamin K2. To do so would be foolish.

I take 1 pill of the Vitamin K mix called "Super K" from www.lef.org for each 10,000 IU's of Vitamin D3 I take, it's just a guess, but I have had no problems over a one year period. Okay? Please do not take high doses of D3 unless you also supplement with vitamin K2! The Super K pill I take with each 10,000 IU's of D3 contains 1000 mcg of K1 (probably not needed), and 1000 mcg of K2 (of the mk4 type) and 200 mcg of K2 of the mk7 type. If you want a really detailed education about the importance of vitamin K2 I highly recommend the book "Vitamin K2 and the Calcium Paradox: How a Little-Known Vitamin Could Save Your Life" – it is really fantastic and after you read this book you will know more than almost any doctor on the subject. It is a major eye-opener!

The main thing I remember from this book is that modern diets cause widespread K2 deficiency, and the K2 is required to keep calcium in your bones and out of your soft tissues. A widespread result of modern day K2 deficiency is that children get cavities and require braces whereas animals and "uncivilized" peoples have perfect teeth, do not get cavities, do not brush their teeth and do not require braces. "Bad teeth" are caused by the jaw bone being too narrow due to lack of calcium deposition during development, thus there are too many teeth for the stunted jawbone-all caused by a K2 deficient modern diet. Crooked teeth and cavities are not natural and not normal in the uncivilized K2 –plentiful world.

Vitamin K2 is available in many health food stores and on the internet. If you are curious about where I used to get my Vitamin D3 and K2 at retail, I got them from the Life Extension Foundation where they have great quality and good enough prices. However, trust me, I am not trying to sell their vitamins, I've taken others as well and they are usually fine. For your convenience one of the readers of this book has set up a website known as www.takeD3.com that contains links to the products discussed here. The website also has some free articles on Vitamin D3 and my previously published journal reviews for free.

If you want really cheap Vitamin D3 and K2 you can get large amounts of high quality bulk powder from a company called Vitaspace where you can get Vitamin K2 powder for $16 a gram which compares favorably with various retail brands that cost as much as $6,200 a gram when they put them in capsules for you! Vitaspace normally sells to vitamin companies who package their powder into pills. You can see all the Vitaspace deals and instructions on how to contact them at www.takeD3.com .

[Newsflash-It turns out that in rare instances some people can be sensitive to too much Vitamin K2 , especially the MK-7 type. If you Google Vitamin K2 and heart racing you will see what some have said. I thought about it and did some research and realized that the symptoms of too much K2 are the same symptoms of a calcium deficiency! Apparently taking too much Vitamin K2 for some people, gets so much calcium out of their blood and soft tissues that calcium deficiency symptoms are induced. The symptoms include heart palpitations and large changes in blood pressure. So just be aware of this possible side effect and cut back your K2 and switch to the MK-4 type if you ever encounter these problems. I have only had one person out of 100 describe this outcome and he was taking 25 mg = 25,000 mcg a day while the most I ever took was 10,000 mcg a day while taking 100,000 IU of D3. (Note-Vitaspace sells only the mk4 type of K2.)

Toxicity

I will add an interesting abstract from Pub Med here that discusses the Vitamin K depletion idea of Vitamin D toxicity for your convenience.

You should read this!!-keep in mind the author does not distinguish between vitamin K1 and K2-on further research I found that it is the K2 depletion caused by high doses of D3 that can be dangerous.)

5.
Vitamin D toxicity Redefined: Vitamin K and the Molecular Mechanism.

Masterjohn C. Weston A. Price Foundation, 4200 Wisconsin Ave., NW, Washington, DC 20016, United States. ChrisMasterjohn@gmail.com

Med Hypotheses. 2007;68(5):1026-34. Epub 2006 Dec

Abstract

The dose of vitamin D that some researchers recommend as optimally therapeutic exceeds that officially recognized as safe by a factor of two; it is therefore important to determine the precise mechanism by which excessive doses of vitamin D exert toxicity so that physicians and other health care practitioners may understand how to use optimally therapeutic doses of this vitamin without the risk of adverse effects. Although the toxicity of vitamin D has conventionally been attributed to its induction of hypercalcemia, animal studies show that the toxic endpoints observed in response to hypervitaminosis D such as anorexia, lethargy, growth retardation, bone resorption, soft tissue calcification, and death can be dissociated from the hypercalcemia that usually accompanies them, demanding that an alternative explanation for the mechanism of vitamin D toxicity be developed. The hypothesis presented in this paper proposes the novel understanding that vitamin D exerts toxicity by inducing a deficiency of vitamin K. According to this model, vitamin D increases the expression of proteins whose activation depends on vitamin K-mediated carboxylation; as the demand for carboxylation increases, the pool of vitamin K is depleted. Since vitamin K is essential to the nervous system and plays important roles in protecting against bone loss and calcification of the peripheral soft tissues, its deficiency results in the symptoms associated with hypervitaminosis D. This hypothesis is circumstantially supported by the observation that animals deficient in vitamin K or vitamin K-dependent proteins exhibit remarkable similarities to animals fed toxic doses of vitamin D, and the observation that vitamin D and the vitamin K-inhibitor Warfarin have similar toxicity profiles and exert toxicity synergistically when combined. The hypothesis further proposes that vitamin A protects against the toxicity of vitamin D by decreasing the expression of vitamin K-dependent proteins and thereby exerting a vitamin K-sparing effect. If animal experiments can confirm this hypothesis, the models by which the maximum safe dose is determined would need to be revised. Physicians and other health care practitioners would be able to treat patients with doses of vitamin D that possess greater therapeutic value than those currently being used while avoiding the risk of adverse effects by administering vitamin D together with vitamins A and K.

End Abstract.

My comment: I would say you might skip the vitamin A –it only suppresses your need for vitamin K2-that's what I did with no harm so far- so rather than suppress the need for more K2-just take more K2.

6.
Megadosing

When I told a third year Northwestern medical student that I was going to boost my dose of Vitamin D3 from 4,000 IU a day to 20,000 early in my experiment she thought I was EXTRA-CRAZY! and warned me of all the dangers I might face from Vitamin D toxicity. My father, a retired Stanford-educated MD, also told me I was "barking mad" and I was going to kill myself in short order! (By the way I have now convinced my father, after the amazing results of my experiment, to take 7,000 IU every day (still too low I believe)). Anyway, if you mention any of this to a normal medical doctor, he or she will highly encourage you not to take the risk. This fear of Vitamin D3 is almost an involuntary reflex that has been ingrained in them from their first days of medical school. You only have to get on the internet and read the writings of Dr. JJ Cannell who is head of the US Vitamin D council, and his words will comfort you as he urges people to take 50,000 IU a day for 3 days at the first sign of a cold. He also thinks the recent increase in the daily allowance for Vitamin D3 from 400 IU to 800 - 2,000 IU a day approved by the US Government sanctioned commission is a joke and almost criminal! He thinks 10,000 IU's should be a good daily dose for most. (I will suggest up to 3X more for someone of my weight (about 200 pounds))- Note added later- I am now thinking after going up high on D3 for a year or so, you should start testing your blood and take just enough to keep your blood levels around 90-100 ng/mL-almost impossible to do without blood testing which you will soon see is cheap and easy and basically painless.)

If you are still worried about high dose vitamin D3, I will comfort you more later, but for the mean time keep in mind and feel free to look up on the internet the 1966 case of a number of pregnant women that wanted to prevent a genetic calcium problem in their babies to be born by taking 100,000 IU a day of Vitamin D for the entire 9 month term of their pregnancies with no ill effects, and completely healthy babies born to boot! (keep in mind this might have been the weaker version of Vitamin D which is D2.)

New information!: I recently received a fantastic email from Mark Murphy! Here is an excerpt from his email-stuff I did not know!

"I believe your doses of D-3 could still be low. The toxicity of D-3 has been greatly exaggerated by Big Pharma and the AMA. It has been researched for a very long time as you know. Evidence of this is the creation of the international unit (to confuse the public) and the manufacture of three prescription drugs Dalsol, Deltalin and Drisdol to fight cancer during the time when the benefits were being rapidly discovered. Dalsol, Deltalin and Drisdol were simply 50,000 iu doses of vitamin D. If there is money to be made, they will try and control us. Look at how much money they have made on the cancer industry.

During the Vitamin D debates during the late 1920's, our government commissioned a nine year study by the University of Illinois, Chicago Medical College on toxicity levels of vitamin D. It is referred to generically as the "Streck Report" of 1937. This study involved 63 dogs and 773 humans. They reported: "There were no deaths among the 773 human subjects whose doses routinely given ranged upward from 200,000 IUs total daily dose for periods ranging from seven days to five years." Also, "One of the authors took 3,000,000 IUs total daily for fifteen days without any evidence of disturbance of any kind."

"Further Studies on Intoxication With Vitamin D" -- I. E. Streck, M.D., H. Deutsch A.B., C. I. Reed, PhD., College of Medicine, University of Illinois, Chicago. Annuals of Internal Medicine, vol 10, no. 7, Jan. 1937" (Keep in mind they used Vitamin D2 which is 1/4th to 1/16th as potent as Vitamin D3).

My "Dangerous" Experiment

Okay, now that we have the history of Vitamin D and it's so called "dangers" sufficiently out of the way for now, let's get down to what you really want to know. What was so miraculous about my self-experiment with ultra-high doses of Vitamin D3? Well, let me get you "hooked" on reading the rest of this book right now:

I at the time of this first writing am 51, but around age 27 I started accumulating injuries and things that just would not heal. Nothing major, but just those nagging things that doctors don't think are serious enough to fix or don't know how to fix, but things that you would like to get fixed nonetheless. At age 27 I didn't realize at the time that the nagging health problems I was and would be accumulating were all likely related. (Oh and later I will tell you about all the other related problems I had as a kid like asthma, ADHD, and scleroderma, as well as the problems of my mother like rheumatoid arthritis, depression, varicose veins, chronic fatigue syndrome, knee replacement surgery, miscarriages and others that were all likely caused by or allowed to occur due to Vitamin D3 deficiency).

If none of that grabs your attention, then consider if you have any interest in possible prevention of obesity, Crohn's Disease, irritable bowel syndrome, ulcerative colitis, diabetes 1 and 2, psoriasis, dandruff, arthritis, autism, (and likely ADD/ADHD), MS, ALS, many cancers including leukemia, heart disease, heart failure, heart hypertrophy, strokes, bronchitis, tuberculosis, other lung problems, childhood schizophrenia (which becomes adult schizophrenia) , COPD and its bronchitis or emphysema, shingles, lupus, any other autoimmune disease, the common cold, alcoholism, ulcers, gastritis, probably-acne, pregnancy complications, allergies, cavities in kids and adults, and many more-including plantar fasciitis & inability of bones to heal due to osteopenia you will still be very be interested in the rest of this book, even if my personal miracles do not impress you. I expect by the end of this short book you should be convinced that almost all the common diseases of mankind that are not caused by inborn rare mutations nor caused by most forms of aging, are ALL likely due to deficient Vitamin D3 levels!

The Amazing Results

So much for theory for now, you probably would like some facts; go ahead and check this out- I hope you will be as amazed as I still am.

- At age 28 I was studying Thai Boxing and doing a lot of kicking with my right leg, this was after my high school and college careers of soccer and rugby where I was also kicking with my right leg quite a bit. At 28 years old I developed a right hip click. I had never heard of it, and thought it was rare. But I think the reason it "seems" rare is because doctors have no good way of treating it. You see hip clicks turn out to be quite common amongst ex- athletes; it turns out many people have them. I have now started talking about it around town, and many people say "I have a hip click too!" They are often associated with sports activity, and there is not a lot that can be done about them. Now if doctors had a pill or a quick surgical fix for it, I bet hip clicks would be as well-known as erectile dysfunction and Viagra! I tried to cure it on my own. I tried deep tissue massages, chiropractors, acupuncture, etc. with no relief, and as I got into my 40's, it got worse and started hurting whenever I walked for more than a block. For about 19 years it didn't hurt, it just made an audible muffled noise when I spread my legs open like they were wings, but around age 47 or so, it started cramping up to the extreme and I would have to stretch my leg or I couldn't walk due to the pain. I finally decided to get serious and try to fix it. I did some research and the medical community suggested they would perform surgery to "relax" the iliopsas tendon which they thought was snapping over the hip. Sorry! I hate surgery, and I looked up how people rated the results for their iliopsas surgery; there were a lot of complaints. I decided to try other things; and then my D3 experiment began. Now, 9 months into high dose

D3, somehow my adult lifelong CURSE of a snapping, painful (lately) hip is 100% GONE! Whatever was causing it, I believe dissolved, because I did go through a number of months of pain in my hip as it seemed to melt and then be healed properly, sometimes requiring several ibuprofen for me to get through the day. I think some sort of dissolving and remodeling process caused the pain, but more on this later. (Was this just a coincidence-as the 3rd year Northwestern med school student suggested?? Check out my next problem-)

- Also around age 29 or so, while studying Thai boxing, our instructor encouraged us to throw elbows at hard objects to toughen our elbows up and make them dangerous weapons. So for a while I would smash holes through drywall with my left elbow, hit the bags all the time and it got a little bigger and bonier on the end. Well that was years ago, and by the time I was 35 or so, I had a large bone spur on the end of my left elbow. A spur is like an additional piece of bone that grows over the original bone. You've probably seen some older men with a real knobby elbow or two here and there. Mine stuck out so much that people made fun of it and my girlfriend's son used to always grab it. It was UGLY! Anyway, during my ninth month into my experiment with high dose D3, I noticed a little pain when I would rest my elbow on the car arm rest, but never thought much about it as it always hurt just a little. So I never checked to see if anything was happening to it until just recently; I looked in the mirror, and the damn thing was gone! At least 90% gone. So maybe my hip click disappearing was no coincidence either, in fact maybe a hip click is actually caused by a bone spur as well- Okay next problem:

- Another thing I got at about the same age (28) was from running around barefoot in the gym shower. My whole prior life as a kid I went barefoot at all pools and locker rooms, and never had a problem. I guess I just thought athletes' feet and foot fungus was something others got. Then one day maybe age 28 or so suddenly I picked up that nasty toenail fungus that gets under your nail and turns it yellow and thick and makes it crack. But you can't get rid of it since it is under the nail. Soon enough all my toe nails were infected. I was told by a pedicurist that the only way to get rid of it is to completely remove all your toenails surgically. Sorry! That sounded too painful!! In later years they came up with a pill that sometimes gives you liver failure, but if it works it takes 3 months of taking these poison pills that will go through your blood and kill the fungus that lives under your toenails. Lamisil I think it's called. I tried it for 5 days and my wrist tendons started hurting so I stopped. I tried it a second time, same thing. My toes still remained an embarrassment. I then heard of laser treatment for $450 with iffy results. I passed. But the laser treatment gave me the idea to heat my toenails up with a magnifying glass in the sun; which I think might work for some people, but my results were so-so at best.

- I then got serious and tried many homegrown remedies to cure the toenails including filing them down and soaking them in bleach, oregano and tea tree oil /apple cider vinegar, etc. I even painted them with Rogaine (minoxidil) which makes nails, like hair, grow faster. I even cut off the thumbs of rubber gloves and put the various treatments on my nails and then covered my big toes with the thumbs of rubber gloves so that the poison would soak in for 24 hours; it didn't really work for me but it seemed clever and might work for someone else. These things didn't work very well for me over a 2-year period. I think just the filing of the nails made it seem like there was some progress by reducing the yellowest outer layer. Oh!, and earlier I also used that nail polish with poison in it called PenLac; that did not work either. And I had filed my nails religiously for 4 months like they suggested and applied the stuff as directed. As you might have already guessed, my dangerous vitamin D3 experiment completely knocked out my yellow nails in about 10 months. Without me doing anything! This also jibes well with my internet research on high dose D3 takers; a number of them said they had yellow fungus under their fingernails that went away with high dose D3. However, most people with the problem of under the nail yellow fungus have it under their toenails and not their fingernails. Why you might ask? I am guessing that toenails almost never see the light of day and thus are especially susceptible to Vitamin D3 deficiency, while fingernails are in the sun all the time. I am now conducting an experiment on my handyman who has the nastiest, yellowest toenails in the world-according to him! I have never seen them but will ask him to take a picture of them tomorrow and start him on 30,000 IU of D3 a day. (Later you will read that he took D3 in high doses intermittently but never consistently) We will see what happens in a year -he is too embarrassed to show them to me!

I now have another case to report-a friend of mine showed me the most disgusting crooked yellow thick cracked toenail you could ever imagine. Luckily for him it was only on his big toe and one other toe. I told him to buy ½ a kilogram of D3 from Vitaspace for $50 and take 20,000 IU a day. It worked alright, about 3 months into his therapy you can see perfect looking baby-like pure toenails half way along- then the remnants of the nasty yellow toenail at the end. I do have a picture of it and will try to post it to the www.takeD3.com website. Unfortunately he had trimmed the worst of it off before I got the picture-but you'll get the idea.

- About 8 years ago, somehow I injured my wrist while carrying large pieces of wood up a ladder. My wrist hurt after pushing wood all day, and when I got home it blew up like a golf ball size swelling on my wrist. It seemed to be filled with fluid. Well it never went away; sometimes it would swell up if irritated and other times with rest it would deflate. After about 4 years I finally broke down and went to the best bone and wrist doctors I could find (a nice perk for being self-insured for medical insurance-which I highly recommend-I have made out handsomely over the years!). They evaluated me and told me I had a ganglion cyst which is like a cyst in your tendon's sheathing that occurs when too much pressure is applied. What happens is similar to getting a weak spot on an inner-tube that bulges out. The doctors tried to remove the fluid; then injected it with cortisone, charged me $450, and said if it didn't get better they could cut it out for $4,000. Having the correct diagnosis, I did a little research on the internet and found these are called "Bible Bumps" because in the past people used to treat them by slamming them with a bible or other heavy book. They would explode under the skin and sometimes heal. I also found out that often the surgery is more painful and worse than the cyst, and it often does not work. Even worse, the cyst often comes back after surgery! So about 3 years ago when it was really swollen, I hit my cyst with a rubber car dent hammer and boom it popped and went flat and the pain instantly went away. But after a few months the cyst came back. Lucky for me, I decided to start my dangerous experiment with high dose Vitamin D3, and now after about 9 months of doses from 20k to 100k, (right now I am stabilized at 25-30k a day), the cyst has hardened and shrunken dramatically. It is not 100% gone yet, but it no longer gets big; it never hurts, and right now instead of being like a fleshy golf ball under my skin, it's as hard as a rock and the size of a pea and still shrinking. (It also seems to shrink more when I take metformin (glucophage is the brand name) - a diabetes drug that lowers your blood sugar but also is supposed to make you live longer-it makes rats and mice live much longer in experiments and makes humans lose weight! You can get it from various online pharmacies without a prescription. Also lef.org is raving about the benefits of metformin and how it prevents all sorts of cancers and should be taken like a vitamin-you can read about it at the Life Extension Foundation website.

- Also around age 27, I got what I later found out was a subcutaneous cyst on my face. It wasn't big, but annoying; it is like a large submerged pimple that never pops completely and continues to flare up from time to time. I went to a dermatologist at age 28 who injected it with cortisone after trying to lance it and expel the contents. (Sounds a little like the ganglion cyst). It didn't work. He told me though, that it is usually seen in older men, but I was stuck with it from a young age for many years until I underwent my "dangerous" Vitamin D3 experiment. The only other "cure" doctors offered me was to use a hollow tube skin biopsy punch to punch out a small hole in the center of the cyst; they then scrape out the "capsule" (they call it) inside the cyst , and scar tissue fills in the space-leaving a lifelong scar. Not pretty. However, finally after a year+ of high dose Vitamin D3 it just one day "popped" on its own. I touched my face and felt a lot of skin oil in the cyst area and realized the cyst had flattened to nothing and finally had given up its ghost! Thank you Vitamin D3!

- Around age 34 or so, I injured myself playing paint ball of all things. Since my girlfriend was playing with all her friends I was trying to be extra impressive, and crawl around, run, duck, and cover, and anything else to impress, and I did end up capturing the flag. However, somehow I injured myself unknowingly, and I didn't find out until the next day when I couldn't lift my arms due to extreme pain in my shoulders. I rested them, but they were never the same; they both clicked and popped like crazy! So much so that a masseuse I had been going to regularly refused to massage them like she used to-it scared her. This condition persisted for years, maybe ten years. I went to the sports doctors for the Los Angeles Lakers, and they X-rayed my shoulders, and told me that I had bone chips in them and they did not recommend surgery since I was not an athlete. They said you're just going to have to learn to live with it! I told them I still wanted to lift weights and things, and they told me, "Well you'll just have to go light." A few years later I went to an HMO to see if they had anything for me, and that Dr. told me I had a torn rotator cuff and prescribed ultrasound therapy. I went for a few month-worthless! The only relief I actually got, believe it or not was from a Chinese Medicine "Witch?" Doctor who magically rubbed my shoulder and transferred his energy into it or so he said, and it actually did feel better for two days, but then again, it went right back to normal-BAD! I gave up! But then I read an article in a magazine (Life Extension Foundation magazine to be exact-you can find them on the web); it was just a brief few paragraphs, and it said that about 80% of the people that complained about bone and joint aches, were found to be deficient in Vitamin D3. After learning this- I immediately ordered up some D3 and started taking 4000 IU a day. I had been getting 400 IU a day in my multivitamin, but apparently that was way too low. What happened at 4000 IU a day? In a month, I kid you not, those many years of snapping clicking hurting shoulders went away. Luba, my masseuse was amazed, and I could work out again without pain or injury. However, only my real obvious injuries were healed. In addition to the shoulders I had been carrying around a lower back injury that I got from arching my back improperly while doing the military press, maybe at age 32. This injury from time to time became excruciating and never healed until recently. It got really bad if I drove for a long time. I got some relief from a chiropractor for the extreme pain, but it would always come back in a few weeks. Well this injury also disappeared in a month after I started 4000 IU a day. So I stayed on 4000 IU a day thinking it was 10X times the recommended dose, and I was pushing the limit! I stayed on this dose for about 6 years. But the hip click, the cysts, the bone spur, and yellow toenails all stubbornly remained.

- Oh- Another thing I figured out, when I was about 6 months into my dangerous experiment I discovered a lifelong idiosyncrasy of mine completely disappeared. Since age 5 or even younger I always had weak and easily sprained ankles, and when I would wiggle my feet I could always get my ankles to crack. I just thought that was normal for me. The weak ankles were never too much of a problem except for the occasional sprain, and when I tried to play ice hockey as a kid, I got good mentally at the game and could be in the right position to steal the puck, but once I got it, the thrill was quickly over as other kids with strong ankles could easily overtake me. You know the weak skating ankles if you've ever been to a skating rink; the kid's ankles give in and his skate blades turn out at opposite directions from each other and it almost looks like the kid is walking on his ankles and not skating on his feet. That was me! Well like I said, 6 months into my dangerous experiment I could no longer make my ankles click after a lifetime of clicking ankles. I also noticed I cannot crack or pop my knuckles anymore!! I am guessing that I have stumbled onto an answer that has stumped doctors forever. Why do peoples' knuckles crack? The only answer I ever heard from a doctor was he said that it was just excess nitrogen escaping the joints. I have another idea...*maybe any joint clicking or knuckle popping you have means you do not have an optimal amount of D3 in your system!*

- One last major thing that seems so easy to forget, I haven't had a cold that has lasted more than a day for at least 7 years since I started taking the 4,000 IU a day dose. While on 4,000 IU a day and more, whenever I got a cold, it just felt like a little under the weatherness that just didn't catch. It went away in a day. I guess that's unusual, but it just seems normal for me now. But I was not always like this. I still can remember those nasty colds with the coughing and wheezing and fevers, and feeling horrible and just wanting to stay in bed for a whole week. The last one of those I can remember was back in the early 2000's.

- Let me just add a few more less miraculous things that I have noticed. At around age 31, I had an injury that occurred while skiing at Steamboat Springs, Colorado where I cut through the woods to get to another trail. I had to ski down a tiny little path and then back up to get through to the next run. Well as it turns, apparently the ski patrol didn't like people cutting through the woods, so right at the lowest point of the path, they had dug out about a pit about 3 feet deep and 4 feet across with vertical walls. I was going too fast to stop; I was either going to crash into it or had to try and jump over it. I jumped as high as I could but my skies landed flat on the opposite wall and really jammed my knees as if I had jumped off maybe a 20-foot building and landed on the sidewalk. My left knee swelled up, and I had to limp for a while. When I got back home I went to the Chicago Blackhawks' orthopedic surgeon and he was going to charge me $800 for an MRI or $3000 to scope it and fix any damage he found. I took a third choice. I decided to limp for a while and see what happened. Well amazingly, it slowly got better, but over the years every once in a while it would grind out of place, click and then swell up, and I had to limp for a week or so. During my 9 months of this dangerous experiment, this knee also started hurting quite a bit along with my shoulders and hip when I initially started taking high doses of D3. But like all my other injuries this one now seems to be completely resolved!

- I am not sure if this is my imagination or not, but right before I started my dangerous experiment, I was getting to the point where I was going to need reading glasses. I found myself, like everyone over 39 or so, having to hold small print further and further from my face to read it. I still have to hold things away from my face to read them, but it seems that this problem is maybe 30% better than before. But since this is such a small improvement compared to the other ones I have experienced, it might just be my imagination. I'll keep you posted on a website that I will set up and/or later editions of this book. (Several months after first publication of this book I decided to begin an experiment of putting Vitamin D3 into my left eye each day for a month (as long as nothing bad happens), to see if it actually can remodel my eye to improve my vision. I will add an update in a later version of this book. At this later time of re-editing I have tried it for only a few days; I have noticed that it just blurs my eye for a little bit after application and this quickly goes away.) Later note- I stopped for no real reason after a week or so-it seemed to be working- but since my overall eyesight seems to be acceptable, I'll wait and will start it again soon and update later-maybe after I go for a period of stopping the D3 for a while.

- Finally, this is not too much of a concern of mine, but it might interest readers who would like to lose weight. When I started boosting my daily D3 intake from 4000 IU to 20,000 IU then even higher beginning about 9 months ago, I weighed about 204 pounds usually. One thing I noticed while taking the higher doses of D3 was that I would sometimes get to working on things and forget to eat all the way until maybe 5pm. Other things I noticed was that when I went out to dinner with friends at the same old restaurants, I would no longer want to finish my normal portions of food and there would be leftovers. My weight came down a little bit, but I hadn't changed my diet in anyway; I still ate cheese pizza very often still drank red wine, had omelets in the morning, and lots of chocolate. After a few months it didn't seem like the weight was changing much; I was stuck at around 197 or so, so I quit weighing myself. Just a week or two ago I thought maybe I would check my weight for fun. I hopped on the scale and it said 179! And I haven't even been trying to diet! I'll let you know if the weight loss continues in a later version of this book. [Oh in case you are wondering –I found that taking 50,000 to 60,000 IU a day really cut my appetite, and I now weigh 179 and am dropping quickly-so possibly the weight loss dose of Vitamin D3 without trying (if I am normal) is 50,000 IU per 200 pounds-or 250IU per pound-but it would be best to check your blood levels, mine were 122 ng/ml after dosing at 25,000 a day I have upped my dose to 50,000 to 60,000 a day for two months-so the weight loss D3 blood levels I'm guessing are around 150 ng/ml.(A later test showed 165) I'll take another blood test soon and update this book for weight loss in the future]. (Oh and another thing I noticed my weight loss really increased when I started drinking 1 quart (1 liter) of 1% milk every morning with a doughnut or pastry-possibly the combination of high d3 and high calcium seemed to accelerate my weight loss-I doubt the doughnut helped.) Also, you should order the 99 cent book on Amazon by Dr. Hollick where he discusses how fat cells can eat up your Vitamin D3 and keep it hidden from your system. This means if one is very overweight and has a lot of large fat cells that he or she might need a much higher dose of D3 to boost their blood levels. (Recently this book was unpublished but can still be read for free at: http://www.naturalnews.com/ SpecialReports/Sunlight.pdf).

A side note: After writing all this out, I started to notice a certain age kept popping up. It was age 27 or 28 or so when I started accumulating health concerns that would not go away. And it got me thinking, what could have changed in my life around age 27 or 28 that might have affected me? Normal aging is one concern, but it did not take long until I realized that age 27 was when I decided to become a 100% vegetarian (with the exception of eggs, cheese and milk-which I could never give up). Before age 27 I used to eat chicken and fish regularly. Quite possibly, cutting fish out of my diet around the age of 27 was a big enough reduction in my Vitamin D3 sources from my diet to trigger the Incomplete Repair Syndrome as I call it. Back then I took a lot of supplements and I still do, but I expect my ingestion of Vitamin D3 was on the lower side, maybe less than 1000 IU a day which caused the problems. End-side note]

Not hooked on D3 yet? Well, let me tell you, I have done a lot more research on D3 and found it likely should help prevent or even cure almost every chronic disease that does not go away on its own that is not 100% aging related or caused by a novel genetic mutation!. And as far as aging goes, taking the right dose Vitamin D3 everyday might also have a large impact on slowing parts of the aging process because as humans get older, their ability to make D3 by exposing their skin to the sun declines dramatically.

But why take my word for anything? I'll tell you. I have been studying aging from the biochemical to the hormonal levels all the way up to the evolutionary level since roughly 1988. I have had 3 relatively-major papers about aging published on the topics; one in 1998, The Evolution of Aging a New Approach to an Old Problem of Biology-Medical Hypotheses Sep 98, and two more in 2000. My 1998 paper caused a bit of a stir and I received reprint requests from 100's of eminent scientists from all over the world and from the best institutions. My next 2 papers weren't as well received since I challenged a major belief that mainstream scientists adhere to, that group selection is impossible-more on this later. I make the case in all these papers and provide evidence that aging is programmed and timed by changes in our hormones that occur with age; no big shock if you understand that hormones drive our whole lives from the cradle to at least menopause. I made the simple jump from this obvious fact to the idea that hormones also cause us to age and die. Simple for you and me, but a radical idea for the mainstream evolutionary biology community.

7.
Aging and Vitamin D3

Wait –before I go on about this, I should add another thing in my past that might be relevant. I have been thinking about aging and evolution and health for almost 25 years now, and always coming up with ideas and theories. One idea I had came after I had been studying the concept of caloric restriction and how it extends life span in all species studied. I simply asked myself- why would evolution want you to live longer if you were in a famine? The answer came to me in that evolution would want to make sure that at least one mating pair of a group was young enough to reproduce after a famine, especially if it was a long one. Otherwise the group would go extinct.

Thus, caloric restriction not only stops the aging process for the most part (and prevents reproduction which could be lethal for both mother and child in a famine)-it actually rejuvenates you (or at least the rats and mice). Well, scientists have been confirming and reconfirming these results many times over ever since the first experiment demonstrated lifespan extension in starved rats in 1933 by Clive McCay as described in the Journal of Nutrition. You can Google this study if you want to. Since then there have been a huge number of experiments demonstrating the life-extending effects of caloric restriction.

Over and over again our scientists like to reconfirm these amazing results. (Seems a bit like a repetitive behavior.)

Well, again I asked myself a simple question, what causes famines? And the answer I came up with is droughts! They are usually longer than famines and precede and cause the famines.

My Methuselah Rat

I then wondered if there is a life-extending evolved response to famine, shouldn't there be a longer, stronger, life-extending evolved response to drought since a drought is longer than and causes a famine?

I then tested this idea on a small group of rats: 2 water restricted rats, and 8 controls (who just lived normally). Amazingly, one of my two water restricted rats lived longer than the longest living calorically restricted rats that I could find in all the experiments on the record! It lived a WORLD-record 47 months!! The oldest CR rat of this kind I could find lived 45 months and there had been 1000's of this type of rat undergoing caloric restriction (basically semi-starvation) to get their one long-liver of 45 months! Most control rats do not make it past 23 months.

I have a little video on YouTube which you can see if you punch   in http://www.youtube.com/watch?v=skLVAQgWx60&feature =youtu.be in your browser. (You can also search for it by typing in longest living rat in the world-I think-in the YouTube search box-it is posted by Jeffbo7777). I add this here just to demonstrate that I have had some luck in coming up with unusual, novel theories that make predictions that when tested are confirmed by the test results!

Interestingly I told the head of the NIH's (=the US Govt's National Institute of Health) Methuselah Project about my water restriction test results (the Methuselah Project is inviting different experiment suggestions to create the longest lived mouse or rat, and then funding the most promising hoping it can be applied to human health). Well, the head scientist who runs the program said basically "Oh that is interesting but we cannot do that experiment because dehydration is bad for you!!" This "scientist" did not care that my rat had set an all-time record for lifespan!! Just the idea of water restriction set off alarm bells in her head since she had always been taught that water is good for you! This kind of proves a point that I will make later in this book about the sorry state of our science community today-run by semi-autistics who get mad if the furniture is rearranged!

Also, I gave these results to multiple scientists in the aging field and they wanted nothing to do with them and only tried to figure out why my experiment should be ignored!!! It was easy for them since my experiment was done at home in a closet and not at a science lab, and I only had two experimental (water-restricted) animals, never mind that one of them set the world record for life span for the rat type in question (Sprague-Dawley females)!

8.
An Alternative / Logical Explanation of Aging

Okay- back to the subject at hand, I was telling you that it seems obvious to us lay people that our hormones could quite possibly be involved in aging us on purpose, but our esteemed scientists cannot accept this idea-

The mainstream evolutionary biology community accepts a theory of aging that says we just all fall apart due to an evolutionary mistake! It is assumed we just "wear out" by living too long because evolutionary biologists have latched onto the simple idea that something that is bad for you could never evolve! Why? Because it would reduce the spread of your genes by limiting the number of children you could have. They believe all of evolution is driven by genes trying to spread further and further and never do they restrain their own spread. This sounds logical on the face, but if you read my papers, you will see it could be a gross oversimplification of evolution. And from my perspective, evolution is a lot more clever and complicated than their simple model can explain, and I map it all out and show how indeed aging can evolve and be selected for by evolution even while being bad for the individual. I won't go into it here other than to say that I DO agree that hormones that are bad for you could not evolve, HOWEVER, hormone patterns that would harm you by accident , could evolve if they occurred at ages you never normally live to in a dangerous environment; they could occur by accident due to random mutations in genes that usually never get turned on. And then when the environment became safe enough for you to live much longer than normal, these accidental hormone patterns/gene expressions that are harmful could make themselves known by aging you. I also go on to show that if these accidentally evolved harmful hormone patterns/gene expressions kill you, but it is good for the group, that evolution can capture them and use them to promote the group's survival even if it is to the individual's detriment. (This might make your eyes glaze over-but believe me –this simple concept is essential to understanding aging-read it again and again until you get it! It is where all our scientists and theorists get hung up and fail! Once you understand it-you will know more than all the scientists out there-assuming I am right-which I am sure I am.)

How could limiting the amount of reproduction by each individual be beneficial to the group? By preventing one individual from fathering or bearing all the offspring of a group, you avoid the trap of having a group of clones or identical twins reducing the group's diversity. In other words, if all individuals were identical twins, and a new predator or bacteria evolved that could kill one individual, it could kill all, and the group would go extinct. Having diversity in the group by preventing (by aging) any one individual from reproducing too many times creates a defense to new forms of mortality causing a 100% extinction by killing all the clones, through introducing enough variability into the gene pool that at least a few members of a population will be different enough from the others to survive a new disease or new predator.

The Riddle of Alzheimer's - Solved?

One indication that my aging theory is correct is that in my 1998 paper I predicted that luteinizing hormone (LH) causes, at very high levels, Alzheimer's disease and any form of organ shrinkage or atrophy or cancers that occur from aging. This huge increase in LH occurs in men and women after age 40 (increases by 1,000's of percent). LH is the hormone that causes the egg follicle (pimple) in a woman to rupture by causing the cells of the follicle tissue to be destroyed, this causes the follicle to burst, which releases the egg, thus making it possible for sperm to reach it for fertilization. The facts are that after age 40, LH levels go way up and get more bio-active and can then attack any tissue in the body-just like it was a follicle! Just recently, 13 years after I proposed this idea, it turns out that the NIH (National Institute of Health) has jumped on the band wagon and put out a paper in 2011 where they implicate LH in causing neurodegenerative disease , and there was another study back in 2002 showed that the most damaged portions of the brain in Alzheimer's victims are full of Luteinizing Hormone which until recently was only known to affect sex-related tissues!

I have added the abstract about the NIH paper to the end notes, but don't get too upset if you don't understand all or any of it, I just wanted to include it here for my own satisfaction since I have received no credit from all the scientists who jumped on the LH / AD bandwagon after my 1998 paper.

If you or a loved one is afflicted with AD you can email me and I will tell you what I know about how to stop its progression (at Jeffbo at aol dot com).. There are some promising ideas that will probably work but you will not hear about for probably 10 years or so while the testing takes place. [Note added later: I decided to write another book that will tell you everything you need to know about how to stop Alzheimer's in its tracks, it is titled-

"Alzheimer's treatments that actually worked in small studies! (Based on new, cutting-edge, correct theory) that will never be tested & you will never hear about from your MD or Big Pharma!"

It contains information on how to stop Alzheimer's and it suggests that to stop Alzheimer's you basically have to stop the aging process-and how to do this. I know it sounds crazy, but read the book and judge for yourself!

Okay I have digressed too long on this point because from what I know now, Vitamin D3 deficiency is more related to our lifestyles rather than aging. But to some extent it is also caused by aging since aged skin cannot generate Vitamin D3 in the sun as well as young skin, but let's leave that point alone for now, and let's pretend that Vitamin D3 deficiency is caused by lack of sun, or lack of taking Vitamin D3 supplements regardless of our age. So how did I recently discover the amazing benefits of Vitamin D3? Let me tell you:

9.
The Dangers of Vitamin D3-Deficiency

Wait, before I tell you, let me tell you a quick summary of all the diseases that seem to be related to low levels of Vitamin D3 based on my reading or browsing of 52,000 abstracts or titles of science journal articles regarding Vitamin D: All of them! Usually from 1967 to 2011 but the Vitamin D titles go all the way back to 1922.

Low levels of Vitamin D3 are associated with or are becoming known to cause the following diseases:

1. Obesity-almost all obese people are deficient in Vitamin D3 and doctors' advice that we started getting in the 1980's to stay out of the sun or use sun screen is what has caused the obesity epidemic we see today! It's not diet or lack of exercise, although these may play a part. Obesity is caused by lack of sun/lack of D3 not by junk food or lack of exercise! Or as I now call it the Human Hibernation Syndrome. If anything, lack of D3 causes you to develop an insatiable appetite for fats and carbs.

2. Depression- seasonal affective disorder (SAD) occurs in winter when our sun exposure is at its lowest. 100,000 IU of D3 has been shown to be way more effective than light therapy for treating SAD.

3. Arthritis-at least 80% of people with bone and joint problems are deficient in Vitamin D3-I bet 100% once they change the definition of deficient!

4. Autism- it now seems the huge increase in autism since the 1980's has also been caused by doctors' advice to us to stay out of the sun, and autistic births have high peak months of March and November when sun exposure is at the minimum, it is also higher in the winter months than summer months, but not as high as the March or November peaks, and this might be explained by the role of snow reflecting sun onto the skin in December through February. This also explains why autism occurrence is higher in northern latitudes than southern attitudes, and in dark-skinned people who need about 6X more sun to create Vitamin D3 in their skin than whites need to create a similar amount (30X more according to the Vit D expert-Dr. Hollick in his 99 cent book Amazon e-book previously mentioned.) Oh and by the way there is an e-book called "Emily's story" that is short, but describes how some autistic kids had a great reaction to high dose Vitamin D3 therapy.

5. MS seems to be caused by Vitamin D3 deficiency and is more prevalent at northern latitudes and almost unknown near the equator.

@@@### newsflash!!!- i just received a youtube link from a reader in brazil for a video about how brazilian doctors are curing – yes, *curing* (as I suspected) MS with high dose D3…make sure you check it out – it is ½ hour
http://www.youtube.com/watch?v=erAgu1XcY-U

---

6. ALS (low D3 levels in ALS patients: cause of ALS or effect?)-Upon further research, I have later found that ALS is more like Alzheimer's and is an age-related disease

7. Schizophrenic babies have low Vitamin D3.

8. Asthma- the incidence of Asthma has been skyrocketing since 1980-low D3 in asthmatics (I had asthma as a child) (I have recently learned that there are several trials going on in the world where asthma sufferers are being given "high" doses of Vitamin D3 to treat asthma.) an additional note-A lady in Alaska who reviewed my book under the name of Alaska Dancing Bear on Amazon-has described how her lifelong asthma has been CURED by taking 20,000 to 30,000 IU a day of Vitamin D3-this led me to write another book for asthmatics which has 6 new pages added to the beginning of this book describing human Lung Remodeling Hormone-at the end of 6 pages I admit there is no such thing as human Lung Remodeling Hormone but that I made it up, and that I was really talking about Vitamin D3!. In the book I also site cases of Dr. JJ Cannel's readers also realizing asthma cures from high dose D3!

9. Scleroderma- a collagen disease-patients have low D3 (I had a benign form of scleroderma as a child)

10. Allergies-Probably dangerous peanut allergies! (I never heard of these as a kid (1970's) -but now they seem quite common!)

11. All minor autoimmune disorders like dandruff, psoriasis, etc.

12. Many types of cancer, prostate, breast, colon, leukemia, pancreatic etc. etc.

13. Tuberculosis

14. The common cold which is much more prevalent in winter months than summer months

15. Toenail (and fingernail) fungus, which a number of people taking high doses of Vitamin D3 have claimed cured their symptoms (including me)

16. Type 1 diabetes which occurs in children when their insulin producing cells are destroyed by the immune system (they all have low D3)

17. Type 2 diabetes which usually occurs in older and obese adults. (all low in d3)) (I will add a very exciting additional idea in the latter part of this book that occurred to me after the initial publication of this e-book-that explains the evolutionary purpose of diabetes and metabolic syndrome as a FASCINATING sub-theory of the Human Hibernation Syndrome!-Stay Tuned!)

18. Metabolic syndrome related to type 2 diabetes-/ insulin resistance).) (I will add a very exciting additional idea in the latter part of this book that occurred to me after the initial publication of this e-book-that explains the evolutionary purpose of diabetes and metabolic syndrome as a FASCINATING sub-theory of the Human Hibernation Syndrome!-Stay Tuned!)

19. Hypertension (I will add a very exciting additional idea in the latter part of this book that occurred to me

after the initial publication of this e-book-that explains the evolutionary purpose of diabetes and metabolic syndrome as a FASCINATING sub-theory of the Human Hibernation Syndrome!-Stay Tuned!)

20. Rheumatoid arthritis

21. Crohn's disease, Irritable bowel syndrome , and Ulcerative colitis (see the dramatic case of Maggie's curing her Crohn's disease of 50 years in the testimonial section at the end of this book.)

22. Alcoholism (thought to be a reaction to depression) and occurs at higher levels in northern latitudes. I have a close relative who was a terrible alcoholic and had not been able to quit drinking hard liquor beginning every day at 1PM for 20 years or so. After about six months of taking a somewhat high dose Vitamin D3, he one day just quit drinking-all on his own and now only has the occasional beer.

23. Ganglion cysts (me)

24. Subcutaneous cysts (me)

25. Acne [Interestingly the Vitamin D3 receptor not only competes with the thyroid-3 (T-3) hormone receptor, but also the retinoic acid receptor, and retinoic acid is used as an acne treatment (and to treat wrinkles) . Getting a tan also is a good treatment for acne which of course increases the Vitamin D3 in the skin in the affected area.]-see the testimonials about how high dosed D3 cured a boy's acne when accutane did not.

26. Heart disease and heart failure/hypertrophy

27. COPD and it's subset diseases of bronchitis and emphysema

28. Lung problems (other)

29. Lupus (see review at end of book from a lady whose skin lesions and sun allergy completely resolved in 7 weeks with 10,000 IU's a day of D3.)

30. Macular Degeneration (one high dose D3 taker claims D3 cured his-see the abstracts) (I will add a very exciting additional idea in the latter part of this book that occurred to me after the initial publication of this e-book-that explains the evolutionary purpose of diabetes and metabolic syndrome as a FASCINATING sub-theory of the Human Hibernation Syndrome!-Stay Tuned!)

31. Growing pains in children

32. Kidney disease ALL have low D3 (I will add a very exciting additional idea in the latter part of this book that occurred to me after the initial publication of this e-book-that explains the evolutionary purpose of diabetes and metabolic syndrome as a FASCINATING sub-theory of the Human Hibernation Syndrome!-Stay Tuned!)

33. Pre-term Births (Preemies) which have gone up 36% in last 25 years. (due to sunscreen? Reduced by ½ in expectant mothers taking 4000 IU of D3 a day (too low I say) (nursing mothers are recommended to take 6400 IU a day. I say too low also!)

34. Small babies, babies with colds or eczema, mothers with infections

35. Pregnancy complications like pre-eclampsia, high blood pressure, gestational diabetes (reduced by high D3 dosing)

36. Miscarriage due to autoimmune attack of fetus

37. Ulcers and helicobacter-pylori related gastritis

38. Death during childbirth

39. Learning disabilities and brain deformities in children

40. Anorexia Nervosa (much higher in March births)

41. Manic Depression-(This one was easy since lack of sleep induces mania, and too much sleep induces depression-this sounds like Vitamin D3 cycling via sun exposure no?)

42. Strokes during and after pregnancy-up 54% since 1994!

43. Strokes in general-a recent study showed a 56% increased risk in stroke in areas with less and weaker sunlight.

44. Non-specific bone pain

45. Excessive daytime sleepiness (see one of the book's reviews-the reviewer claimed a cure!)

46. I am going to add ADD and ADHD here because as a child I had asthma as well as ADHD, and recently I learned that kids with ADD or ADHD also are highly susceptible to asthma. While I have found no studies yet suggesting the link between maternal Vitamin D3 deficiency and offspring with ADD or ADHD, I believe it is just a matter of time until this link is

found. Additional weight given to this connection can be found in the fact that some of the genes involved in triggering autism are also involved in triggering ADD/ADHD. And since we know that autism is linked to low maternal Vitamin D3 levels we can pretty much take a wild guess that low maternal D3 also causes ADD/ADHD in offspring.

47. Glaucoma-Dr. Kaufman of the Glaucoma Institute has discovered that Vitamin D3 drops put into the eyes of monkeys reduces their intra ocular pressure by 20 to 30%!,(Wait until they feed them 30,000 IU day!!) (I will add a very exciting additional idea in the latter part of this book that occurred to me after the initial publication of this e-book-that explains the evolutionary purpose of diabetes and metabolic syndrome as a FASCINATING sub-theory of the Human Hibernation Syndrome!-Stay Tuned!)

48. Migraine headaches-see abstracts at end of book.

49. Parkinson's disease (Outdoor workers have lower incidence of PD)

50. Urinary Tract Infections

51. PMS

52. Menstrual cramps-see last abstract

53. Gout-it turns out high uric acid levels eat up your Vitamin D3 or low D3 causes Gout

54. It just dawned on me that since various psychological/psychiatric conditions have been found to be associated with low D3 levels, two more

conditions seem quite likely to be caused by low D3 also. Hoarding Behavior/ and it's associated/somewhat similar condition- OCD (obsessive compulsive disorder). Why? If evolution is preparing you for winter famine when your D3 levels are low, it seems quite logical that you might start hoarding all sorts of things including food!

55. Cavities in teeth and especially baby teeth! Just saw a report on the news that cavities in children's teeth are way up. So decided to look it up and many sources, including Dr Cannell-Head of the Vit D institute, described how giving kids just 1,000 IU a day of D3 stopped the formation of cavities

56. PSORIASIS-Now this is amazing! You can read the review of my book at Amazon by Donn Carroll an MD-Ophthalmologist who had lifelong incurable Psoriasis so bad that he had to sleep on his stomach. After two months of 50,000 IU a day- he was completely cured and "On Top of the World!".

57. Plantar Fasciitis-I had this for about a year but it went away before my big experiment- while I was taking just 4,000 IU a day. I have been informed by a reader from Brazil that he had plantar fasciitis for two years and started taking 25,000 IU a day and it was gone in 2 weeks!

58. Osteopenia-Another reviewer recently wrote about how high dose D3 and K2 caused a broken bone in her foot to heal after 6 months of failure following her Doctor's advice.

59. Vertigo Plus Migraine-A reader recently emailed me from Scotland that high dose D3 quickly cured her recently acquired migraine combined with vertigo.

60. Chronic wounds and ulcers that will not heal-Read the email I recently received from a lady with a chronic wound that would not heal until she started taking 75,000 IU a day of D3 posted at the end of the book.

61. Knee Degeneration Requiring Knee replacement-I just received an email from a reader whose doctors were telling her she needed both knees replaced. After taking 2,000 Iu of D3 for 60 days and upping the dose to 10,000 IU for a month more she claims her knees are now completely fine. See her email at the end of the book.

62. Near/Far sightedness-the same reader with the knees above also noticed that her eyesight had improved from +2.25 to .75 in her right eye and +.75 to -.25 in her left eye (whatever that means) and her eye doctor's assistants asked her if she had corrective surgery. See the email at the end of the book. (I also noticed that my far vision has seemed to be getting clearer, like looking into deep water that used to be a bit cloudy and now it seems as if it is crystal clear and depth perception is much more pronounced-but I wondered if it was just my imagination. Given that D3 remodels various tissues it seems quite possible that it remodels the lens of your eye as well.

63. Actinic keratosis-A red haired/fair skinned reader says he has suffered from a lifelong condition Actinic

keratosis where exposure of his skin to the sun causes thick scaly patches of skin to develop of which have a 20% risk of turning into cancers. See his email at the end of the book.

64. Sunburn- Apparently some people who burn easily do not burn while taking high dose D3..see last email end of book.

65. Bone spurs- My bone spur on my elbow disappeared in 9 months with high dose D3 , and a recent email I received was from a man who had two bone spurs on his ankles that were the largest his podiatrist had ever seen. He had had them fro 20 years. Gone after 26,000IU a day of D3 for a number of months-see email at end.

66. Severe Hypoglycemia/Hypogonadism- The most remarkable email to date from a man who had suffered terribly from severe untreatable hypoglycemia since a child. Cured in a month! The high dose D3 treatment also boosted his testosterone levels to the point were at age 25 he started growing a beard for the first time in his life.

67. Varicose veins-No kidding I have been seeing people blogging about watching their varicose veins shrinking down to look like little spider webs while on high dose D3.

68. Incontinence-the mother of the reader who set up the takeD3.com website for us has a mother in her 70's who had a hard time holding back her urine and would have to run to the bathroom and would often

have accidents. After about six months taking 10,000 IU a day she no longer has the problem.

69. Infertility-It was found that 93% of women who were infertile were Vitamin D3 deficient-See the testimonial at the end of the book from a lady who failed three attempts at In Vitro Fertilization and only succeeded after taking 20,000 IU of D3 a day for a few months. (It would make sense that evolution would make one infertile if it anticipated a winter famine around the bend to prevent one from losing resources to reproduction that were needed first for survivial.)

After reviewing this list, a number of readers who write AMAZON reviews (usually Amazon hyper-reviewers) say something like "If it sounds too good to be true, it usually is". Or "health claims overblown". To them I say, before you speak, learn and read; if you go through all 52,000 studies done on Vitamin D3 to date (now 55,000) on Pub Med, it will only take you about 3 to 6 months, and you will then speak from a base of knowledge rather than from a base of beliefs.

Anyway, some people just have the need to spout off and let everyone else know what they think they know. What I have learned from these reviewers is that common sense is not so common! Did they not read that I have looked over 52,000 studies regarding Vitamin D? I guess they missed that, or did not understand what that means. Anyway, I just don't want someone to miss a cure for this or that because they focused on someone regurgitating their conventional wisdom that sounds so logical on its face. The list of diseases related to

D3 deficiency above <u>is</u> correct. Most of the list is indicated from the study of the 52,000 abstracts, while there are just a few that are anecdotal accounts from readers.

10.
I Believe Anyone Can Find
A Cure For Any Disease
in 30 Days or Less!

I haven't done this yet, but you could educate yourself some more by just typing in "season of birth" OR "month of birth" in the Pub Med database and reading all the titles of the 3,600 science journal articles that come up, and you can probably guess that many of the observations will ultimately have something to do with maternal vitamin D3 levels during pregnancy.

Now, what about osteoporosis?? Common sense would tell you that if D3 is good for your bones a D3 deficiency should cause osteoporosis. I believe this is not true! I searched the Pub Med science article database that goes all the way back to 1967 and earlier.

For the search terms "D3 deficiency causes osteoporosis" from that search I only got 79 hits ! If D3 deficiency actually caused osteoporosis we would have had at least 1,000 hits! Sure-I have seen the studies that suggest low D3 levels lead to increased fractures, but this is not , I believe from osteoporosis, which can also cause increased fractures, but rather more likely from poor bone maintenance. I can guarantee you and almost bet my life from the abstracts you will see if you do a quick Pub Med search that D3 deficiency does not cause osteoporosis.

I mention that here and show the results so that you can get used to doing your own searches and answering your own questions in Pub Med. You really don't have to know anything to start. You can just dream up a question, and if it is true, you will get a lot of results specifically saying it is true. And you don't have to read the whole abstract. Most of it is just a lot of numbers concerning the experiment. Each abstract has a title, and introduction, and a conclusion. Just focus on the title, and introduction, and a conclusion for a while and soon, even without any education in a field, you will start to see a pattern. Patterns usually mean something and lead to other questions. I believe most people could cure any disease just with Pub Med database research in about a month! No kidding!. All the scientists out there seem to be just churning out little puzzle pieces from their little area of expertise, and almost nobody is working on the puzzle! In fact if you look at the all the science journals out there, you will find that about 99% of them deal with results of experiments or clinical observations. I only know of one medical journal devoted to theory-Medical Hypotheses! That should tell you how dysfunctional our science community actually is! I believe most scientists are borderline autistics that love repetition, sameness, and are generally pedantic (enjoying correcting others) and, like autistic children , they get mad when the furniture is rearranged! It seems all the creative people go into the arts or film, or writing novels, and for some reason none of them make it into science. That is why the Pub Med database just sits there with all the answers we would ever want for all diseases, just waiting, just sitting there, undiscovered! All for the lack of a creative person working about 30 minutes or at most 30 days on a disease!

You can freely access the Pub Med database on the internet and do your own thought experiments by going to this address: www.ncbi.nlm.nih.gov/**pubmed**

Since so many experiments have been conducted since 1967 and reported to Pub Med, if you construct a question and type it into the search box and it is false, you will get a way smaller number of hits, and the hits will generally be something only peripherally related to your question. So, the results I got from my question"D3 deficiency causes osteoporosis" (it's not really a question- call it a hypothesis) , you will soon see, suggests that D3 deficiency does **not** cause Osteoporosis (You can learn a lot just by figuring out how databases with huge amounts of data work!) I've been doing this as my primary form of research for more than 25 years- so believe when I say there are easily observed patterns in the data that will give you answers-It just takes time, like doing a jigsaw puzzle.

Later note- a recent study was publicized on the news suggesting that Vitamin D3 supplementation (very low dose) with calcium did not help women with osteoporosis-just as my theory would predict. However they did not use a high dose so maybe the dosing was the problem. Until higher D3 dose studies are done, I am extremely comfortable saying I am right. They also suggested the calcium supplements caused an increase in heart disease due to calcification. I am sure they did not give these women vitamin K2 to keep the calcium in their bones and out of their blood, veins and soft tissues! Their final advice from the study was a criminally negligent "Do not take Vitamin D3 for osteoporosis"-and completely ignoring the multitude of beneficial effects that D3 has on everything else! I saw a recent suggestion from someone that this misinformation- study was put out as a first step in trying to outlaw Vitamin D3 by Big Pharma!

The bottom line is that the 79 Pub Med results agree with my previously published papers where I suggested that osteoporosis was not caused by any deficiency in hormones but by the *huge rise* in Luteinizing Hormone that occurs in both men and women after age 40. Where LH attacks the bones (osteoporosis), the brain (Alzheimer's) and many other parts of the body.

Basically, it seems that all diseases known to man, other than some of those caused by aging, are all related to D3 deficiency which I call the Human Hibernation Syndrome (HHS) along with its sub syndrome – the Incomplete Repair Syndrome (the IRS). [Oddly IRS is also the acronym for the US Government's dreaded tax collection agency (the Internal Revenue Service)- so from now on when someone notes that they were crippled by the IRS-it may take on a somewhat less ominous meaning than it has had up to now!]

You see I was vaguely aware of the benefits of Vitamin D3 about 8 years ago when I learned that most people with joint aches and pains turned out to be deficient in Vitamin D3. That was when I upped my dose from the standard 400 to 1000 IU a day to 4000 IU a day and I thought that was a high enough dose to give me some good effects. And it did! It got rid of a lot of my arthritic problems that I had been experiencing from age 30 to 39, and I was able to work out again and not sustain injuries to my shoulders or wrists whereas I had been struggling for 10 years to try and work out like I had in my 20's.

Then one day, a big clue came when my father, a Stanford educated medical doctor (MD) / urologist, had been taking at my suggestion 2000 IU of D3 a day for several years finally was given a Vitamin D3 blood test-which he loves to say cost $380 and was paid for by Medicare! (Where I can get an over the counter home test done for $60! (Actually I later found out just $44 from Life Extension Foundation).

I was shocked when my father got his test results back he was still at the very low end of the Vitamin D3 spectrum with 30 ng per ml at age 79! It's best to be over 70ng/ml or so, and some say it is safe up to 150 ng/ml! (I am not sure if 150 ng/ml is safe over long periods and would only recommend going up that high to reverse some problems you might have, and then stabilize yourself around 90-100 ng/ml). His daily dose of 2000 IU at the time was 5 x the recommend daily dose of Vitamin D3 recommended by doctors of 400 IU per day! It was then I thought that maybe I came from a family that has low Vitamin D3 levels maybe caused by our genetics. He had been taking 5x the daily recommended dose, yet he was at the critically low level of 30 ng/ml! (or that possibly the entire medical community has been very wrong for years as to how much Vitamin D3 we all need to take (or how much daily sun we need!)

11.
The Best Blood-Testing Option

The cheapest and most convenient way I have found to get my blood tested in the US is to use the blood test service at Life Extension Foundation we have set up a link to the blood test at www.takeD3.com. It's really easy; you go to their website, select the Vit D blood test, pay them only $44 and they email you a prepaid blood test form. Print it out, and whenever you feel like it take it over to the nearest blood test center (usually Lab Corp) in your neighborhood (they give you several nearby centers' addresses on your form) - probably 5 minutes away! They painlessly take your blood as soon as you get there, then you leave; they overnight your blood to LEF; you get your test results via email in 2-3 days!- I prefer this to paying $60 to stick my finger and squeeze out 4 drops of blood-ouch!) (Also one doctor recommends that you get your blood tested for Vitamin D in the winter when it will be at its lowest. Who cares if you are normal in the summer, it is the low levels that make you sick.)). Maybe LEF provides testing in other countries also-I know they sell products worldwide.

The 4000 IU a day I had been taking for six years or so was enough to prevent my workout injuries, but it had no effect on a condition I had had for 20+ years called a hip click which is often a sports-associated injury, where something goes wrong in your hip so that when you spread your legs far enough you hear and feel a muffled but audible click in the hip. I had tried many ways to fix it other than surgery.

Surgery was suggested by surgeons as the best treatment to relax the Iliopsis tendon so that it no longer caused the clicking sensation by snapping over the bone. Chiropractors really had no idea what to do.

I had read that among other things that hormone Vitamin D3 is the bone and joint remodeling hormone. So after the news of my father's low D3 levels even when supplemented with 2000 IU a day I decided to try an experiment, to increase my D3 dose dramatically to see what happened.

I boosted my dose from 4000 to 20,000 IU per day: 50X the doctor recommended dose! Considered very dangerous if you asked any doctors who had learned about Vitamin D toxicity in their first year in med school.

The initial results were very interesting. I kind of went into a testosterone like mania for a while and had lots of energy and anger-[this is not too surprising since Vitamin D3 is a steroid hormone, a seco-steroid hormone to be precise-which means it is the same shape as a steroid hormone but has one open ring-the second one, where steroids have all four rings closed in a circle].

But I also started feeling pain in all my joints that had ever had an injury before.

I chalked the pain up to the idea that all my old injuries that had never healed properly before were now being dissolved and remade in the proper way- bone and joint remodeling!

I remembered the experiment where they broke the leg bones of rats and saw how well the break healed. The rats with no Vitamin D3 supplements had bone repairs with a large callous on the break, whereas D3 supplemented rats had perfectly healed bones with no callous.

I continued with the 20,000 IU a day assuming the bone and joint remodeling hypothesis was correct, but in the mean time I had to take ibuprofen from time to time to overcome the pain! I also rubbed the painful joints with Ibuprofen cream. And I limped and hurt for a few weeks. Also, it felt like someone had hit my shoulders with a sledge hammer!!

My shoulders hurt, from old rugby and newer paintball injuries. My knee hurt from an old skiing accident, and my hip click was killing me, and my wrist hurt where I had a ganglion cyst that never had gone away for the last 5 years.

Well after about 2 months most of the pain went away, and I noticed my ganglion cyst was hardening and shrinking in size. It seemed to be working! My bones and joints were being remodeled, apparently your body never forgets what the correct bone and joint configuration is, it seems to be just restrained from repairing things completely due to a fear of using up critical resources during winter.

My shoulders still hurt and still hurt now, 6 months later (this part was written 3 months ago) but the main pain is in my left shoulder where I had a rugby injury at age 21 where my shoulder dislocated and I had to have repair surgery at that age. My right shoulder is almost pain free, and my hip click has totally gone away!! The last of the remodeling seems to be going on in my left shoulder which in my 20's had been dislocated in a rugby injury and had been corrected surgically but still apparently had not healed properly. As I write right now, my left shoulder is the last injury to be completely resolved (now at 9 months into the experiment, after going up to 100,000 IU a day and then stopping due to pain, and then going back on 25,000 IU a day, my left shoulder is now completely pain free). However, when I bench press right now, with heavier weights I do feel the left shoulder joint sliding about as if it was kind of jelly like and flexible, not like a hardened stiff bony joint. I expect that after I reduce my dose of D3, that my flexible joints will harden once again, hopefully in the proper repaired configuration of my youth.

I know for sure that my right shoulder has undergone a dramatic transformation since I used to be a pitcher and third basemen in high school and could throw things really far or really hard. In my 30's my right shoulder was so stiff I could not throw a ball out from home plate past second base. But now, when I play fetch with my dogs, I can throw the ball again, three times as far! And my dreams of being a major league pitcher have been rekindled!! -just joking about that.

For a while I had boosted my dose up to 100,000 IU per day but got nervous when I thought or imagined that my kidneys were hurting (I had a test for kidney damage which I mention at the end of my writing), so I stopped for a while for about 4 weeks, and then started again with 50,000 a day which I continue to take at this writing. (Later note, 50,000 caused pain in my joints after a while, I stopped again , and now have been on 25,000 a day for 2 more months- and everything seems perfect). Further note-after 25,000 seemed good I boosted it to 30,000 IU a day where I remain. (It has been about 2 months now at 30,000 and I notice just a slight rise in pain in my left shoulder, and in my right hip where the hip click used to be. I guess there are still a few finishing touches my body wants to complete! [A later writing- I finally decided to boost it up to 50,000-60,000 a day for the last two months to try and get rid of all my pains, the right shoulder hurt for a while-it is completely healed, the right hip click is long gone but the hip still has some minor pain but it is almost gone, and the left shoulder is getting better but is not yet pain free-and I am losing weight without trying-I now weigh 179-and have lost 25 pounds without even trying!].

After the pause and then taking 50,000 a day for a month or so, I started back into that testosterone like mania for a while where political events got me really angry and I started sending out a blog every day to everyone I knew, that semi-rage has subsided after about 2 more months.

You will be happy to know that I researched this as well as I could by reading all 52,000 abstracts or titles of science articles that mention Vitamin D that have been published in science journals since 1967 (some back to 1922) in Pub Med. You too can review all these abstracts by searching for Pub Med on Google and selecting any of the Pub Med website/ search engines and just typing in Vitamin D (no need to trust me!)

To put it simply, what I discovered from all this research is that there is a good chance that Vitamin D3 deficiency is the cause of most of human disease-caused suffering other than aging!! And that all the new epidemics we have been experiencing like autism , obesity, asthma, (maybe ADD) and many more since the 1980's are all due to our following doctors' advice to stay out of the sun and use sunscreen and not to take too much Vitamin D3 since it is dangerous! I'll tell you what is dangerous-Doctors' advice! Sorry Dad!

Okay let me reiterate the logic from an evolutionary perspective as to why this might be true. It is actually amazingly quite simple and easy to follow. All you have to do is ask yourself:

Why would evolution want to you to become obese and depressed if you are not exposed to sunlight for a long time??

Answer: If evolution detects little sunlight, it expects you are going into winter which is the time of a long famine and lack of food and resources. In other words it wants you to hibernate to some extent, just like a bear before winter. It wants you to eat like crazy, and put on many pounds, so a Vitamin D3 deficiency is like a signal to your whole body that famine is coming which will give you carbohydrate and fat cravings among other things.

It also wants you to stay at home and not waste much energy. Thus it makes you depressed...

You might also think that to keep you at home in bed, it wants you to get sick (there is an alternate idea for this later). It also gives you asthma which keeps you home.

It might also want your joints to hurt so that you don't travel much and burn energy.

(Alternatively it also might not repair you completely to conserve resources for the coming famine) Maybe both are correct.

It might also assume that there will be very few resources available for a long time, so that rather than repair you completely which takes more resources, it repairs you just enough to get by hoping you will see the sun again which will tell it that more resources are coming, and when that happens it can repair you fully at a later, safer date.

So again, you see we have come up with a simple concept that Vitamin D3 deficiency causes the Human Hibernation Syndrome and its subset of the Incomplete Repair Syndrome- "the dreaded IRS"!

Well I checked on the internet to see if anyone had come up the idea of the Human Hibernation Syndrome, and I found someone had patented the use of T3, the active form of thyroid hormone (like Vitamin D has a D1 D2 and D3 , for thyroid hormone there is a T2 T3 T4 etc. But T3 is the active hormone, the others need to be converted into T3). This patent suggested that to combat what they called something like the human hibernation syndrome that T3 should be liberally prescribed. What amazed me was that all the diseases that T3 was supposed to conquer pretty much lined up with all the diseases that I was proposing that D3 was to conquer!! I then knew then I was onto something!

So I then looked into T3 vs. D3 and found the two hormone receptors and hormones often compete with each other and sometimes ½ a D3 receptor pairs up with ½ a T3 receptor, and that when you raise one hormone in the body the other goes down! And the T3 and D3 hormones are very similar in structure.

This led me thinking that maybe T3 was the winter version of D3, and tempered the human hibernation response and incomplete repair syndrome but was not as effective as D3. This seems to be the case. They give people with low energy, depression, obesity T3 to rev them up and they often feel better. You can do the same thing by giving them D3 which will also repair them unlike T3.

Interestingly, I looked up hormone changes in bears when they hibernate, and most of the research dwelled on thyroid hormone and its changes. It was suggested that thyroid declined a little while the bear was hibernating, but it wasn't much. I then searched for bear hibernation and Vitamin D3 and found an obscure article that noted that bears Vitamin D3 levels drop from 22 in the summer down to 8 when they are hibernating! It seems bear hibernation researchers have been barking up the wrong tree! D3 is the anti-hibernation hormone, not T3!

I have a handyman who was diagnosed with low thyroid hormone in 2001. He has been taking T4 (not T3) for all these years. His body still has to convert the T4 into the active hormone T3 as needed, but it had helped him. One day he came in to work with an eye infection and I suggested he take a large dose of D3 to see if that would help his immune system knock it out. He started taking 20,000 IU a day, and after 3 days, the D3 knocked out his eye problem (or maybe it was just coincidence and it cured itself) this was after the doctor prescribed antibiotics which had no effect. He kept on taking the high dose for a while.

He described the side effect of this high dose of D3 as to making him feel better than he had in 20 years! He was super-charged with energy and I noticed after he had been taking it for a few months, that his big bear of a body started to shrink and he now only has a pot belly attached to a relatively normal frame. Before he looked like a huge Wooly mammoth, since he is very hairy and has long hair and a long beard, and that used to be his nickname unknown to him! He swears by it now, but I think he is not taking enough, or quit taking it, since he still weighs 240. Maybe I will see if he will experiment more with it before this book is done and I will tell you the results. Or I will tell you in a later edition.

Now let me try to explain in the view of what we have discussed what is going on in the health of the public these days.

Right now we have the first lady Michelle Obama starting a war on obesity in the US public school system. The plan is to eliminate fattening and high caloric foods and get the kids to exercise more. (The Obama administration has also recently enacted a 10% tax on tanning bed sessions assuming they are bad for you-it turns out that some tanning beds can actually dramatically boost your D3 levels especially the UVB beds (vs. UVA).

Well, let me and any older person who went to grade school before the 1980's reminisce a bit and think about our classmates. I can guarantee you that nobody had any fat kids in their class in the 1970's except for maybe one or two-right? If I'm wrong then this theory falls apart. I'm willing to gamble that almost all were like me and my classmates , thin, and we ate all the fattening junk food that we wanted, and there were just a few fatties maybe 2 or 3 in a class of 25, like Mimi J******, and Scott B**** but everyone else was thin! And I also remember that Mimi and Scott were excessively pale (a sign of low D3??) (Oh and I forgot to mention we were almost all of the white race).

When I went to my girlfriend's daughter's 6th grade class in the 2003 to participate in a parent activity I was shocked! She was one of the only skinny ones! Maybe there were 4 or 5 others. The rest were ALL FAT even the boys! About 80% or so of the class was fat!! Many in the class were of Latino background and recent immigrants to the US, at least their parents were, and this jibes exactly with warnings for Vitamin D3 levels for people with darker skin. Darker skinned people who have recently moved north to the US, are at especially high risk for Vitamin D3 deficiency, and thus you see very high rates of obesity in recent immigrants to the US that come from strong sun countries near the equator. This is caused by darker skin needing a lot more sun than white skin to produce the same amount of Vitamin D3! And nowadays I hear that many black mothers are slathering their kids in sunscreen! This is an outrage in my opinion.

Maybe I'm jumping to conclusions based on a small sample size, but you learn in statistics class that a random sample of 30 is usually pretty accurate-and there were more than 30 kids in that class I visited. So what could be the difference between then and now? Maybe now the kids get less gym class and too much computer and TV at home, but I remember all my friends watching tons and tons of television and eating only junk food when I was a kid and we just didn't get fat! We played outside a lot but we didn't use sunscreen-it didn't exist back then-thankfully!

If diets and exercise aren't dramatically different enough to account for the weight differences that we see in kids before and after the early 1980's, what is so different between then and now? Let's take a wild guess! The introduction of sun screen and sun avoidance into American society around 1980!!

(also the ground zero date for the huge outbreak in autism and asthma as well).

It turns out that it is likely our well-meaning physicians in trying to protect us from that evil disease called non-melanoma skin cancer, have created an iatrogenic (caused by doctors) epidemic of obesity, autism, and asthma among many other things. And it turns out that non-melanoma skin cancer is relatively benign and the dangerous form of skin cancer is melanoma which is now being shown to be prevented by Vitamin D3 or sun exposure!

Yes, doctors may have saved a few of us from benign (not dangerous) forms of skin cancer, but they have unleashed a huge epidemic of all the diseases I mentioned earlier and probably more we will find out about later. They gave us diseases by keeping us all out of the sun and telling us to slather ourselves with sunscreen whenever we sneak out into the deadly outdoors for just a minute! Just watch the news these days, whenever it is sunny, the weatherman always reminds you to make sure to wear a hat and put on sunscreen! This is totally wrong advice if you think of the history of mankind and how we evolved mostly around the equatorial regions in very strong sun.

The results of my likely lifelong Vitamin D3 deficiency

So let me tell you now about my life history, and how a lifelong Vitamin D3 deficiency might have affected me.

I was born long before sunscreen was to come into vogue; all we had was tanning lotion or cocoa butter! Remember that Coppertone girl with the dog tugging on her swimsuit and exposing her tan line? I sure do, that was the beach/sun environment we all grew up in. I used to play outside in the sun, and tan with my parents at home and on the beach, and in the summers I was always quite healthy. Both my parents were always working on a good tan when they could, tans were in style then and they looked good and made you look (and probably feel) healthy!

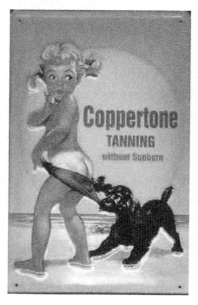

But at about age 4, in the winter, all of the sudden I came down with severe asthma. I remembered that I felt like I was drowning and could not breathe, and my mother and sister would try to help me, but they could do nothing; it was agony, and I still feel sorry for other asthma sufferers even though I haven't had it since about age 6. That's how bad it was! That I still remember it all these years later -maybe it was like water boarding!

Well I was "cured by the doctors" who decided I was allergic to feather pillows, and needed my adenoids out (some sort of tissue behind my nose and in my throat). They cut out my adenoids, and gave me synthetic pillows, and that seemed to do the trick. However in retrospect, since asthma and allergies are strongly associated with low Vitamin D3, D3 supplements or a trip to Florida probably would have also likely done the trick.

At age 23 I moved from St. Louis to Chicago and all of the sudden I came down with seasonal allergies which I had never had before. They started whenever I saw that white fluff from trees or plants floating around in the air. I got pretty bad allergies where I would sneeze continuously and my eyes would itch and tear uncontrollably. I would have to take anti-allergy medicines for about a 4 week period. Eventually I would take Claritin, but always tried to take as few pills as possible. This went on my whole life after I got the allergies. The first year into my D3 experiment I found my allergies were less and only had to take about 5 Claritins. This year-the second year of my dangerous D3 experiment I got through allergy season with 0 Claritins! I am almost cured! I had a few bouts of sneezing when the fluff was in the air-but no need for Claritin. I can thus hypothesize that high dose D3 over a long time will CURE allergies. Apparently it takes a bit longer to remodel your immune system than a bone spur or hip click!)

Also, around age 10 or so I got an embarrassing bald patch on my head. It kind of looked like a saber had cut my scalp from my cowlick down towards my face. We had it diagnosed, and it turned out it was a non-fatal form of scleroderma. Scleroderma is a disease where your collagen misbehaves and does not create proper tissues in a certain area-weird right? In people with the fatal disease, it is like it starts somewhere on their body and it cuts through their entire torso, and when it gets to their heart it kills them. Luckily for me it was scleroderma morphea which just stops at the scalp and leaves a bald spot which I have had my whole life but it has been reduced by a plastic surgeon who just cut pieces out of it and sewed my scalp together and tighter. Well, I did a little research on scleroderma on Pub Med and viola! All the victims are deficient in Vitamin D3. I wish I had known this when I was younger! The doctors did their best at the time and shot my head full of cortisone-seems like a recurrent theme in my life.

Some of the studies I have seen suggest there is a U curve for optimal Vitamin D3 levels, where too little and you get sick, and too much is also bad for you. My guess is that there is an optimal maintenance level, but if you want to heal a number of accumulated unhealed problems, you might want to risk going up the high side of the curve for a while until you have healed your problems and then come back down. Keep in mind, healing yourself under a doctor's knife, or with dangerous drugs is also definitely risky. So I would not be too scared of taking a few risks to knock out some medical problems that the doctors have not been able to solve. I believe my proper maintenance dose of Vitamin D3 is 25,000-30,000 IU a day. Whereas many Vitamin D3 experts often say that 10,000 IU a day can be considered safe, but my guess is they are just being overly cautious as they always are. (And if you listen to common run of the mill doctors who are about 10 to 20 years behind the times they will tell you 2,000 IU is the upper safe limit!) Eventually that recommended level of 2,000 and 10,000 IU a day I believe should and will rise. So, if you weigh about 100 pounds and want to try the course of Vitamin D3 therapy that I have taken you would start off with 10,000 IU a day for a while, and then if you want to heal some injuries boost it up to 25,000 IU a day, then stop when you feel too much pain, and then maybe even a few weeks at 50,000 IU a day, and then later taper off to a 10,000 a day maintenance dose. So make sure you adjust your D3 intake to your weight, and if you are 400 pounds you might want to double the dose that I take until you get down to 200 pounds then cut it in half.

Later note- what I just told you about dosing is wrong if you have the luxury of testing your blood for Vitamin D3 from time to time. In this case, how much you take is completely irrelevant, the important thing is what your blood level gets to! And you all will be happy to know that I finally did break down and test my blood for D3..I will tell you my levels shortly! (A later note- you probably can reduce the risks of high dose D3 therapy by taking high dose of Vitamin K2 when you super dose with D3 which is discussed elsewhere in this book). And I initially suggested you use the home testing kits which you can find on the internet for $60, to keep track of your D3 levels but I eventually switched to using Life Extension Foundation's more accurate cheaper service.

I also recently read Dr. Hollick's excellent 99 cent 24 page e-book where he is interviewed about Vitamin D3. He notes that obese people have a very hard time boosting their D3 levels because the fat cells act to sequester the D3 and prevent it from becoming a circulating hormone. So if you are overweight, you might need to take much higher amounts of D3 to achieve the same blood levels of D3 than a skinny person needs to take. So who knows how much you should take if you are overweight? Any overweight person HAS to have their blood tested at reasonable intervals to get their levels in the 90-100 range otherwise it is complete guesswork and possibly dangerous.

Also, I should tell you about my mother's lifetime experience. Her whole life she hated fish, and most fish is a good source of vitamin D3. So it is no surprise in her older age she suffered many illnesses now apparently related to low levels of Vitamin D3. She had both her knees replaced due to Rheumatoid Arthritis. She often suffered depression. She suffers from weight gain. She has had varicose veins and two miscarriages. (And she had a child with ADHD-ME!) I have warned her many times to boost her D3 levels. But she often never listens to me.

Interestingly, if you look up the history of cod liver oil, it has long been used to treat arthritis, and prevent birth complications, and used to be something that mothers forced their children to take every day for health. Also what is interesting is apparently the doctors of the past realized that living in a sunny climate had health benefits and often when they were unsure of how to treat a patient would tell them they had to move to the south. Often moving south would cure people of their diseases. I just add this here to suggest that even when totally ignorant of what was actually happening at the biochemical level, doctors of antiquity did notice that cod liver oil and moving south had major health benefits. We now know that the benefits are from increased Vitamin D3, but you wouldn't know it if you listen to the current medical establishment's hysteria over sun and skin cancer where they tell you to avoid the sun and use sunscreen. Even the old remedy for diseases of going to health spas, like the Dead Sea, was actually effective. Everyone thought the salts of these old seas were healing them, but rather it was the exposure to sun that boosted their D3 levels that did the trick. So even though I like to pick on doctors from time to time, we should take our hats off to those of the past who prescribed sunshine and cod liver oil to their patients-They were way ahead of their time! (At the time of updating this latest edition, I just heard on the radio that a study just showed that people who live in less sunny (Northern) climates have double the risk of stroke than those who live in sunny climates!)

Now keep in mind, I am white, 5' 11" and about 190 pounds (was 200) (now 179 at a later writing), and the doses that seemed to be good for me were 25,000 of most of the time, and 50,000 IU for a while and 100,000 IU for a short time. Every time I increased my dose I felt pain in my joints with old injuries, but most of the pain was at 25,000 IU for a few months. When I went up to 50,000 IU after 25,000 IU it no longer caused pain; I dealt with it pretty well but then the pain increased. But I kept going, and I decided to go up to 100,000 IU a day since the pregnant ladies I mentioned earlier could handle it. The 100,000 IU didn't cause my joints much pain, but I thought I started feeling pain in my kidneys. So I stopped the 100,000 IU at this point , waited for a while and then went back to 25,000 IU a day (now 30,000) where I remain. At times I almost could not stand the pain in my joints being repaired but I went ahead with it and am glad I did. A good maintenance dose for me now seems to be 25,000-30,000 IU. It turns out that a good level for me for weight loss was 60,000 IU a day which I now at the latest update of this book, continue to take. (Three months after the last sentence was written I completed my final three month experiment of 60,000 IU a day-tested my blood D3 levels and they were at 168 (which is considered dangerous by those who think we should expect to live forever since it increases the risk of atrial fibrillation from 5% (in normal people over age 65) to 12.5% in high dose d3 takers whose blood levels exceed 100.) I then cut my D3 level down to 5,000-10,000 IU a day for a month and retested; my D3 levels came down to 115, will test again soon. Additional information-the three months at 60,000 seemed to do some more repair work to my left shoulder and right hip, but no other joints, as they both hurt during the therapy and for about 2 months after I stopped taking the 60,000 a day. Finally after 2 months after stopping the 60,000/day, the pain is gone and the joints are hardening up and soon I will start heavy lifting again.)

One side effect I noticed, especially when I hit 50,000 IU a day and more, was that I could just sleep like a log for maybe 14 hours. It was a feeling like you get when you have been in the sun for a long, long time, it just exhausts you. Many people who have always used sunscreen will <u>not</u> know what I am talking about. But older people who used to go to Florida on vacation as a kid and would play on the beach unprotected from the sun for maybe 8 hours a day will understand. Expect to sleep a lot when you go high on D3! (Later I found out that taking large doses of melatonin at night, pretty much counteracted the excess sleep requirement which at first seemed a little odd to me since I had earlier experimented with high dose melatonin which also made me sleep about 14 hours a day when taken alone). You see melatonin is made at night when you sleep and is destroyed when you sit in the sun. It also goes way up in animals about to hibernate. So you might call it the winter hibernation health hormone! Thus, taking melatonin and D3 together might actually counteract the healing properties of D3 taken alone. I'm just guessing here, but it seems logical. However, both D3 and melatonin are known to be very good for you so maybe after you heal yourself with high D3, you can then add melatonin to maximize your health situation. A good dose of melatonin for maximal health might be 75 mg for women which has been used in Europe for birth control. A man might adjust it higher based on his weight. I take 120 mg when I am using melatonin (that will be another book in itself as it took me 4 months of sleeping up to 14 hours a day to get used to high dose melatonin, but after a while you can eventually get back to sleeping 7 hours a day). The other interesting thing about melatonin is that it goes way up during caloric restriction (CR) and is likely the hormone change that curtails female reproduction during CR. Caloric restriction is good for you because it basically stops the aging process as much as possible and has been shown to increase mouse lifespan by 20% to 40%. (Another hormone that stays elevated during CR is DHEA which I have taken for a long time now and recommend it to everyone, but it's best to do your own research. You can get good quality info at the Life Extension Foundation just type dhea into their search box and they have most of the information you need. (Again-I am only a customer of LEF and have no commercial or any other connection with them other than admiring their website, vitamins and blood testing.-Other places might be just as good, I am just too busy to look for them.)

An interesting side note

I have started hearing from others who are now taking higher doses of Vitamin D3, and one really neat side effect two others have mentioned to me is that they now find themselves having really VIVID and detailed and long dreams! AND the best part is that the dreams usually involve them visiting with long lost old friends and or deceased loved pets, etc. And when they look at them in the dreams it is just how they remember them even if they last saw them 20 to 30 years ago! And almost all the dreams are really pleasant! Well, how about that? That is exactly the same thing that has been happening to me for the last year-pleasant dreams visiting old friends of the past as well as my old pets. I even had a dream about my childhood cat whom I can't really remember what she looked like if I consciously try; the last time I saw her was more than 30 years ago, but in the dream it was just like I had seen her yesterday as a kid- 100% familiar! Oh well, let us know if it happens to you. I wonder what the evolutionary purpose of such dreams would be if everyone is affected the same way?

12.
Testing your Vitamin D3-levels yourself

If you are more meticulous than I was, you can order Vitamin D3 testing kits that you can perform at home, by taking a little finger prick of blood and mailing to a testing center. Most people have Vitamin D3 levels in the 20 to 30 ng/ml range, while optimal levels are (they say) are in the 70-90 ng/ml range or higher and it is said Vitamin D3 toxicity does not kick in until 150 ng/ml range or more. So if you are excessively nervous about experimenting with your Vitamin D3 levels, you can use these test kits as training wheels. I however, have always trusted how I feel when I am taking something. If I start to feel something unexpected, then I cut back. I will test blood levels soon and report the results in a later edition of this book.(Later note-it is a good idea to test your D3 levels at every step in your therapy and keep it at 80 to 100!)

GREAT NEWS! MY BLOOD TEST CAME BACK..AND-

I recently received my blood test back for the Vitamin D3 levels in my blood and it as 120 ng/ml – the same as Florida lifeguards who do not use sun screen. This after my year long experiment and my stabilizing my maintenance dose at 30,000 IU a day for a few months. The test also noted that I had NOT damaged my kidneys as my Cystatin-C levels were in the normal range. (A later D3 test had me as high as 168.)

13.
Why Sunshine is not
Quite Enough

So if you take a high dose of D3 what is the sunshine equivalent? This is what should give you the courage to try and take higher doses of D3.

Did evolution really design us to only get 10 minutes of sunshine a day and expect optimal health? That sounds ridiculous. Humans not too long ago in evolutionary terms lived near the equator and got lots of sun every day. And one would guess they ran around almost naked. I would guess if sun exposure makes you produce a health hormone one might expect that evolution would want you to get <u>at least</u> an hour a day of strong sun, especially if you lived around the equator. And if you migrated away from the equator and moved north, evolution would have to set up all sorts of compensating adjustments to overcome the lack of sun in the winter (like T3?) . And that compensation is probably still evolving since many of us get sick from lack of sun still.

14.

How to Determine the Right Dose

If we just let our D3 deficiencies go with no D3 supplementation and let evolution take its course, maybe in 10,000 years all the kinks will have been worked out and D3 supplementation might not be needed by future generations that live in the northern latitudes. But until then, I would rather short circuit evolution's selection process as it applies to me and pretend I live at the equator year round by taking 25,000-30,000 IU of D3 a day which is equivalent to just a ½ hour of equatorial sun per day. That doesn't sound so crazy does it?? And over time I might boost that dose if I feel and learn that it is safe, or even reduce it depending on my results. Right now I just don't know the exact optimal dose for me and it might vary for every person depending on their skin color, size, weight, and background, etc. The best way to do it is to check your blood levels regularly and shoot for a target number. I think 120 ng/ml sounds great! (Later note-rumor has it that one researcher (cutting edge) suggests that one should keep one's D3 level at 100ng/ml or less to prevent a possible increase in the risk of heart arrhythmias where your heart beat temporarily gets off pace. While an adult over 65 has about a 5% chance of getting a heart arrhythmia in his or her remaining lifetime, the new research suggests this risk may increase to 12% in people with Vitamin D levels over 120 ng/ml-but I'm not scared (famous last words?) Actually another person I know in charge of a huge blood testing center has looked at the data and has not found this correlation. Just thought it best for you all to have all the facts! Just after writing this new paragraph, LEF magazine reported that those who take fish oil supplements on a daily basis can reduce their risk of arrhythmias by 90%+. So it seems smart to add the suggestion that if you decide to take high dose D3, in addition to sharply upping your daily Vitamin K2 intake, that you add fish oil supplements to the regimen as well. I personally take 6 MEGA EPA/DHA (omega-3) soft gels everyday which costs about $8 a bottle for 120.

I became a little concerned about the increased incidence of atrial fibrillation occurring in people with D3 levels over 100-120 so I did a little research. I discovered that warfarin which is a drug (actually rat poison) they give people at risk of blood clots. It prevents clots by inhibiting Vitamin K1 which helps for blood clotting but it also inhibits K2 which can prevent afib I believe. It turns out that warfarin users have a high incidence of atrial fibrillation (due to K2 inhibition) (even though this is a drug to prevent the bad effects of afib like stroke by inhibiting K1's clotting) which suggests that both warfarin and high levels of D3 both can trigger atrial fibrillation by eating up your Vitamin K2! So make sure you take Vitamin K2 if you decide to conduct this experiment on yourself!

15.
Vitamin D3 Deficiency and Cancer

Interestingly, Vitamin D3 deficiency has been implicated in all sorts of different cancers.

This now does not surprise me since I have read many times that cancer is not a disease of mutation per se, because they say many cells go cancerous in every body's body all the time. The cancer cells are usually destroyed by one's immune system so that cancer is actually a disease of the immune system and nothing more. It is just that your immune system no longer picks up the signals of a cancerous cell and it thinks that the cell belongs to your body. Maybe under the effects of low D3, your body is in famine mode and does not want to kill any cells that might not be able to be replaced. Given that Vitamin D3 supercharges your immune system, then it is not surprising that many if not all types of cancer seems to be triggered by low Vitamin D3 levels.

Autophagy

To add weight to this idea, I did come across a science article that suggests Vitamin D3 boosts the process of autophagy which is roughly the cell body's practice of "self-eating" and might be the important factor that causes Vitamin D3 to have such a preventative effect for cancers, due to the possibility it boosts your body's ability to destroy defective cell organelles and defective cells and tissues in the process of rebuilding them.

16.
New addition to the Human Hibernation Syndrome Theory

The evolutionary purpose of diabetes and metabolic syndrome and their associated symptoms of high blood sugar, insulin resistance, increased blood pressure, and elevated cholesterol:

Diabetes

After writing this book, I just kept getting a nagging feeling that I had missed something important about how diabetes and metabolic syndrome fit into the whole scheme of things. Why? Because obesity, and Type II diabetes and metabolic syndrome occur together so often that I reasoned if obesity is just evolution's way of preparing you for a winter famine, then diabetes and metabolic syndrome must be preparing you for something bad to come as well.

Also, so as not to forget about Type I diabetes which usually occurs in children when their immune system destroys their insulin producing cells in the pancreas- a recent Scientific American article Feb-2012 notes that Type I diabetes is increasing quite dramatically all over the world showing the similar increases as those in obesity and other modern epidemics. Researchers do not know why and wonder if it is caused by some sort of virus or infection! (Likely lack of sun). The end result of both types of diabetes is the same: excess sugar in the blood.

I then started wondering about blood sugar. What in the world could increased blood sugar protect you from? And then it hit me! I remembered some experiments that were conducted on a (poor) Beagle where they wanted to put the dog into suspended animation with no vital signs and then see if he could be resuscitated. They did this by reducing his body temperature to about freezing. In order to prevent freezing damage to his tissues, they added a large amount of glycerol to his blood. This lowered the freezing point of his blood so that they could reduce his body temperature dramatically and not worry about crystallization damage. I also remembered this is what they do to people's bodies who have signed up to be frozen upon death with hopes of being resurrected in the future after technology advances make resuscitation possible (good luck).

Aha! Possibly high glucose levels in the blood protect the hibernating body from the danger of tissue damage due to freezing! By boosting the sugar level of blood, it reduces blood's freezing and crystallization temperature!

With this thought in mind a started looking up what happens to animals while hibernating. Wouldn't you know it?-frogs, amphibians, and insects fill their bodies with glucose and other sugar-based antifreeze compounds and are able to be frozen solid and then come back to life with the next thaw! And then I remembered that car antifreeze (ethylene glycol) is dangerous to cats and dogs because they like its sweet taste and often drink it. Antifreeze is also added to Gatorade (also sweet tasting) by murdering spouses and nurses in many true crime shows on TV!

So then I looked up the hibernating bear. Well the theory didn't seem to hold up so well as the hibernating bear's blood sugar didn't seem to go up so much in the winter. But then I ran across an interesting study that showed that if a hibernating bear ate a small amount of food, he had a huge spike in blood sugar that stayed elevated about four times as long as a normal bear. It seemed like I was onto something!

Now here is the neat part. I started wondering about the parts of the body most damaged by diabetes: the feet-often leading to amputations, the eyes-often leading to blindness, and the kidneys-often leading to kidney failure. I wondered if these organs and tissues were the ones most likely to be damaged by freezing temperatures. The feet made sense since they are the first to get frost bitten. And the eyes are filled with aqueous humour which takes a long time to be replaced-thus there is relatively little heat-giving blood flow going into the eyes! The kidneys seemed to be at risk also since they would have a pretty high amount of non circulating urine building up in them which would also result in making it more difficult for warmth-giving blood to keep the kidneys properly heated. The thought came to mind that maybe evolution has figured out a way to concentrate glucose in the feet, the eyes, and the kidneys in order to protect them from freezing damage if a huge cold snap were to arise.

Well I decided to think of some other body parts that should also be affected disproportionately by freezing, and of course the fingers and the ears come to mind.

So I looked up diabetes and fingers and found that diabetics often do also get their fingers amputated due to damage from diabetes. And although the evidence was scarce, I did find a website for parents of diabetic children where they discussed how diabetic kids' ears would often get swollen and red and they didn't know why!

I then checked to see what parts of the body are most damaged by freezing and of course found feet, hands, ears, and the corneas of the eyes, but there was nothing much on kidneys. However after further searching I found a case of a man who suffered severe hypothermia after being submerged in an icy pond for quite some time while rescuing his dog. Three days after the ordeal, which the doctors thought he had survived unscathed, he had complete kidney failure!! The plot as well as the blood seemed to be thickening!

Finally, I checked out another prediction that one could make from this theory-that Eskimos (Inuit Indians) who live in the cold and would be extra likely to require freezing protection should have a high susceptibility to Type II diabetes and metabolic syndrome-and indeed this proved to be the case.

So, after this crazy brainstorm of several days, I am relatively confident in stating that Type II Diabetes (and likely Type I) as well as metabolic syndrome evolved as evolution's way to protect hibernating humans from the possibility of freezing damage of the most vulnerable tissues and organs. And, while this condition might be temporarily protective, if it persists, the excess sugar being sequestered in the freeze-vulnerable tissues eventually damages them through cross linking reactions.

(Oh and as far a the increased cholesterol goes, it is found that hibernating bears have double the amount of cholesterol and triglycerides in their blood as non hibernating bears due to their living off of fat as opposed to carbohydrates and proteins). Might it also be possible that blood with high levels of cholesterol is less likely to freeze?

Does this idea bring us any closer to developing a better treatment for Type II diabetes and metabolic syndrome? Maybe. Possibly increasing one's body temperature via sauna, or hot tubs might trick the body into thinking that a freeze is no longer a big risk and then blood sugar levels might be reduced. However, the best bet of all is to make the body think it is no longer hibernating which can be done by losing all one's excess weight and then supplementing with vitamin D3 or engaging in sunbathing or tanning bed sessions. Adding daily exercise would also help the body think that the hibernation is over as well. This is nothing new, however, as doctors have long recommended weight loss and exercise as a cure for type II diabetes and metabolic syndrome. However, the addition of Vitamin D3 might make the weight loss much easier by curbing one's appetite. Also, I recently saw a study that increased Vitamin D3 alone actually reduced Type II diabetes and metabolic syndrome to some extent. I have also been hearing from some readers that after about 6 months or so of high dose D3 they are being able to reduce their Type II diabetes medications.

Now wait a minute! What about increased blood pressure? How does that fit in to this theory? I looked up what happens to liquids that are under increased pressure, does it lower their freezing point?? I was almost heartbroken-no! Actually increased pressure pushes the liquid molecules more closely together and allows them to freeze at a HIGHER temperature. Well I was about to go back to the drawing board and then noticed this one little caveat...

"Water however, is an exception. Because water increases in volume when it becomes ice, increasing its pressure (while not allowing it to expand) will LOWER its freezing point to some extent." Thus we can explain the increase in blood pressure that many humans endure as an artifact of protection against freezing that evolved in our ancestors!

Viola-it seems all the ducks line up in a row... Is the case closed for now? Seems like it is to me!

[A later update-It was pointed out to me by a high school physics student/whiz kid from Germany in an email that the phenomenon of increased pressure reducing the freezing point of water only occurs at very high pressures-at about 50 times (50 bar) the regular atmospheric pressure of 1 bar. Thus it was impossible to be an important factor at pressures found within one's veins and arteries which are almost never more than 2 bar. But I was sure it had to be right somehow. I then remembered when I put an unopened coca cola in the freezer for a while in a plastic bottle and then opened it to let the pressure of the CO_2 out, the liquid would instantly turn into a frozen slush. Upon further research I finally found that increasing the pressure of water that is in the presence of carbon dioxide (like human blood) forces a lot more carbon dioxide to dissolve in the water and it can lower the freezing point from 32 degrees F to as low as 20 degrees F. So this is why you can cool an unopened bottle of Coke or soda water down to 20 degrees or so without it crystallizing into ice. Once the bottle is opened, the $Co2$ escapes and the freezing point of the liquid shoots up and boom instant ice. This lowering of freezing temperature of water and blood is quite significant and can be the difference between life and death if you were caught out in the freezing cold for a prolonged period.]

Wait. One last thing-I recently heard on the radio that the local government was adding beet juice to the salt it puts on the city streets in the winter to prevent icing. Beet juice is sweet, full of sugar, and then it hit me-SALT! Yes salt lowers the freezing point of water and is often added to ice baths to reduce the freezing temperature of water from 32 degrees F to -6F in a completely saturated solution of salt water. And then I remembered that many people are told by their doctors to reduce their salt intake especially if they have high blood pressure. The doctors see a cause and effect where there is none. It has never been proven that high salt intake causes or increases hypertension. I think there is another explanation-if you have low D3 levels your body thinks you might encounter a freezing period and thus causes you to crave salt-so you eat more salt. Salt <u>does not cause</u> high blood pressure, <u>it works with</u> high blood pressure to keep you from freezing. And I then looked up salt craving and yes indeed it is found in people who are Vitamin D3 deficient. Maybe we should rename type II diabetes and metabolic syndrome-the Human Antifreeze Syndrome?

[One last insight has recently popped into my mind. The Vitamin K2 content of food available from an animal's environment varies quite a bit with high levels being found in the tissues and milk of animals that graze on grass during the summer months. If these animals are food sources for humans, humans' Vitamin K2 levels will likewise have a seasonal variation. The K2 level drops quite a bit in these animals during the fall-winter-early spring season. So when you are at the organic food store and see various foods such as meat, butter and milk advertising that they came from grass-fed animals, you now know why food products from grass-fed animals are considered to be so healthy. If the animals are raised on corn like most animals are, they do not produce any Vitamin K2. And if you look at the butter in organic food stores advertising that it is from grass-fed cows you will also notice they usually add that the butter was harvested in the summer months. Again this is when the K2 produced is at its highest and one can even see it in that the butter is a much more orange color than winter harvested butter.

How does all this fit into the Human Anti-Freeze Syndrome? If humans evolved in environments where the levels of Vitamin K2 varied dramatically in their diets between summer and winter, humans would be depositing calcium into their soft tissues (veins) during the winter months when K2 was low and reversing the process in the summer when their K2 levels were high. So we generally think of calcified arteries and veins as a bad thing and in modern humans it is. However it is possible that calcified arteries and veins have a much lower freezing /crystallization point and thus our ancestors may have survived freezing temperatures of winter by temporarily calcifying their veins and arteries during the winter and de calcifying them when the K2 levels rose in their food sources in the summer which then caused the veins and arteries to lose calcium and have it put back in their bones. This idea could be tested with a few simple experiments, and if true it would be a simple matter to reverse atherosclerosis and a many effects of heart disease with high dose Vitamin K2 supplementation.

NEW INFORMATION ENCOUNTERED AFTER THE FIRST WRITING OF THIS BOOK:

Boost your testosterone levels with Vitamin D3?

I recently saw an ad for a book by Dr. John Cannell who published a book titled: The Athlete's Edge: Faster, Quicker, Stronger With Vitamin D,

Here is what Dr. Cannel says about his book: "This book covers new ground. After extensive investigation and translation of numerous scientific reports into the English language, author Dr. John Cannell reveals a long-held secret once known only to Eastern European athletic trainers. In the 1960s and 70s, it was called Sunlamp Therapy, and it gives athletes a definitive edge over their competitors, particularly for athletes who train for indoor or winter sports. That vitamin D, the sunshine vitamin, improves muscle tone, muscle strength, balance, reaction time and physical endurance, as well as immunity and general health, is a recent discovery in western medicine. It has application ranging from improved performance of standing armies in the field, to Olympic and every-day athletes, and even seniors who need to avert falls and age-related loss of muscle mass and muscle tone. This ground-breaking book is a welcome addition to our current working knowledge of nutrition and health. Read it from beginning to end."

In an ad for Dr. Cannel's Vitamin D3 formulation it is written- "The roster of Vitamin D's researched benefits is growing almost faster than scientists can get the word out. And now, testosterone support has been added to this exciting list. In a landmark study, 3332 IU of Vitamin D taken as a daily supplement for one year raised testosterone levels in Vitamin D-deficient men."

If Vitamin D3 actually boosts testosterone levels in those who take it this then might explain the kind of "roid rage" I seemed to be getting when I initially boosted my Vit D3 dose to 20,000 IU a day. It might also explain why some readers of my book have noted in the Amazon review section that higher doses of D3 have acted somewhat like a Viagra-like aphrodisiac!

And finally, a young man, 26 years old, who had suffered sever hypoglycemia and hypogonadism (low testosterone) his whole life , experienced a dramatic rise in his testosterone levels after just one month of very high dose Vitamin D3 therapy.-See his testimonial at the end of the book.

17.
Differences between Vitamin K1 and Vitamin K2

The second interesting new point I have come across regarding Vitamin D3 concerns the differences between Vitamin K1 and Vitamin K2. A recent article put out by the Life Extension Foundation titled 'Avoiding the Catastrophic Event" summed it up very nicely. (This was an article where they detailed why Jack Lalane-who was doing everything right- died of aortic stenosis at age 95 when everyone expected him to live to 300!). It turns out Jack didn't know about Vitamin K2! Had he known, age 95 would have been just a minor speed bump on his superhighway to immortality.

It turns out Vitamin K1 is what you need so that your blood will clot and you get it in your diet from leafy green vegetables and it will convert minimally, and not easily, into Vitamin K2. (The differences between Vitamin K1 and K2 are so great that some suggest renaming them to avoid the confusion.) (Later Note- I recently read an article at the Vitamin D Council website that suggests Vitamin K1 DOES convert pretty easily to K2).

Vitamin K2 can also be found in cheese, egg yolk, butter, chicken, salami, ground beef and natto (a nasty fermented Japanese dish). Eating a lot of most of this stuff is unhealthy so you are better off getting your K2 from a supplement.

So earlier in the book I warned that you should take large doses of Vitamin K with any high dose Vitamin D3 regimen. That is what the recent journal article suggested where it said Vitamin D3 toxicity has the same symptoms as Vitamin K deficiency, but the author did not differentiate between Vitamin K1 and Vitamin K2 in the abstract. It turns out that we need to take extra Vitamin K2 with high dose D3. Why? Because high levels of D3 apparently go about repairing your bones and joints. To do this it needs to enlist the help of a calcium regulating protein called matrix gamma-carboxy glutamic acid (we'll just call it MGP from now on). MGP either inhibits or promotes calcification based on its state of carboxylation. If carboxylation is too low, MGP causes the arteries to calcify and it prevents the repair of your bones and causes your bones to lose calcium with which it calcifies your veins! When MGP is fully carboxylated, it inhibits the calcification of your veins and arteries (and decalcifies them) and sends the calcium over to promote the repair of your bones. K2 is really amazing. Make sure you get it.

So how do you carboxylate your MGP? It requires Vitamin K2! That's it. If you don't get enough K2 you might calcify and die! Vitamin D3, in repairing your bones and joints, eats up MGP like crazy- eventually giving you a K2 deficiency with all its dangers. So to get the wondrous results of high dose D3 without the disastrous results of D3 toxicity- all you need to do it seems is supplement with Vitamin K2. And that's what I did and I am still alive. For every 10,000 IU of D3 I took, I also took a "Super K" vitamin from lef.org that contains 1000 mcg of K1 and 1000 mcg of K2 of the MK-4 type and 200 mcg of the MK-7 type. (MK-4 comes form animals sources and is a bit shorter acting while MK-7 comes from bacterial sources and is a bit stronger. You can get MK-7 from Natto.) I recently switched to Vitaspace's Mk-4 Vitamin K2 as it is a lot cheaper and supposedly the form of K2 that is free from heart racing side effects in a few people (more on this later).

18.
Obesity

Just for fun you can go onto the internet and Google a map of the US that shows obesity by state. You will see a general trend of obesity increasing the further north you go. There are however, huge exceptions, like in the deep south. After viewing the obesity map, you can then Google a map that shows relative concentration of African Americans by state. You will see that most of the weird results where you have high obesity in high sun southern states are caused by having a high percentage of African Americans.

Why? Because their skin requires anywhere from 6 to 30 times the amount of sun that white skin needs (depending on who you believe) to make the same amount of Vitamin D3 as whites!

Some Readers are Sharing Excellent Additional Information

I recently received a fantastic email from Mark Murphy. Here is an excerpt from his email-stuff I did not know. "I believe your doses of d-3 could still be low. The toxicity of d-3 has been greatly exaggerated by big pharma and the AMA. It has been researched for a very long time as you know. Evidence of this is the creation of the international unit (to confuse the public) and the manufacture of three prescription drugs Dalsol, Deltalin and Drisdol to fight cancer during the time when the benefits were being rapidly discovered. Dalsol, Deltalin and Drisdol were simply 50,000 iu doses of vitamin D. If there is money to be made, they will try and control us. Look at how much money they have made on the cancer industry.

During the vitamin d debates during the late 1920's, our government commissioned a nine year study by the University of Illinois, Chicago Medical College on toxicity levels of vitamin D. It is referred to generically as the "Steck Report" of 1937. This study involved 63 dogs and 773 humans. They reported: "There were no deaths among the 773 human subjects whose doses routinely given ranged upward from 200,000 IUs total daily dose for periods ranging from seven days to five years." Also, "One of the authors took 3,000,000 IUs total daily for fifteen days without any evidence of disturbance of any kind."

"Further Studies on Intoxication With Vitamin D" -- I. E. Steck, M.D., H. Deutsch A.B., C. I. Reed, PhD., College of Medicine, University of Illinois, Chicago. Annuals of Internal Medicine, vol 10, no. 7, Jan. 1937"

I need to add a note here that they were likely using the less active form of Vitamin D which is vitamin D2 which comes from irradiating plant matter with UV light. It is thought to be form $1/4^{th}$ to $1/16^{th}$ as active as Vitamin D3 in humans- thus if we divide all the doses noted above by 4 or up to16 we should get an activity-equivalent level for D3. Thus for example, a person taking 3 million IUs of D2 in a day might get the same effect as taking as little as $3,000,000/16 = 187,500$ IU's of D3 or possibly as much as $3,000,000/4 = 750,000$ IU's of d3 depending on which conversion ratio is correct.

Finally, while the hard copy of this book will likely not be updated except in rare instances, any eBook version of this book will be updated probably monthly as new information comes in. So, if you are interested in staying current you might like to purchase the cheaper eBook version of this book from time to time.

19.
Different qualities of
Vitamin K2

WARNING! WARNING! WARNING!!! I recently read n the review comments section of my Amazon book site that some people had been experiencing racing hearts when they took Vitamin K2. But also the writer had found a quote from someone on the internet that when he switched brands of K2 that his heart racing went away. Here is what he said: it turns out when he switched from Jarrow's to LEF's K2 his symptoms went away. I am guessing that there are some manufacturing issues that a number of suppliers have not figured out yet. It would be best to stick to LEF's K2 for now I would say (maybe even better to use Vitaspace's pure Mk-4 type of K2 at $1/100^{th}$ the price-go to www.takeD3.com for Vitaspace's info.). Here is his quote:

"I dare say most of you have read this in the previous thread, but just in case here it is again. (I was suffering horrendous symptoms, my heart was all over the place and hearing my heart beating in my ear all the time was very disconcerting. My doctor was very concerned and told me to stop jogging and referred me to a vascular consultant. This consultant could find nothing wrong. At first I did not associate my vitamin K intake as being connected. I put a message on this site and someone replied and told me that she had had heart arrhythmias which stopped about a week after she stopped taking vitamin K.

I had taken vitamin k because, 'Reading that natto was so beneficial in promoting bone and cardiovascular strength, I began taking Jarrow Formula's vitamin K2 as MK-7 (derived from natto). I was taking one a day (90 mcg), but began to suffer severe arrhythmias and pulsatile tinnitus.' I stopped taking all vitamin K and sure enough within a week my symptoms stopped. 'The only vitamin K2 MK-4 I could find was Life Extension's Super K with advanced K2 complex. Each gel capsule contains 1000 mcg K1, 1000 mcg K2 as MK-4 and 100 mcg K2 as MK-7'. I started taking these expecting my symptoms to return BUT, 'Surprisingly, although these contain slightly more MK-7, since I have been taking these I have had no occurrence of arrhythmias and the tinnitus has vanished!

It doesn't really make any sense! I wonder if anyone else has had a similar experience.

I live in the UK and had to get the vit K shipped from America'. Will follow LynH's advice and try Amazon in the future.

I think this site is wonderful as I have received such knowledgeable help. Most of you are so much more informed than most doctors! Thank you so much to everyone."

My note- I think I finally figured it out-see the symptoms of calcium deficiency that follow. Apparently in a few people, too much K2 or too strong K2 causes so much calcium to be removed from the blood and soft tissues and put in the bones that calcium deficiency symptoms occur-but this is rare and easily reversed.

Calcium Deficiency Symptoms in Women

Mar 28, 2011 | By Lori Newell

Calcium is essential for strong teeth, and it plays a role in making sure the heart beats correctly, the muscles contract, blood vessels dilate and relax and many other functions. For women, getting adequate levels of calcium helps keep the bones strong and prevents osteoporosis. Since so many foods contain calcium, a well-balanced diet should supply the daily requirement of 1,000 to 1,200 mg. If calcium levels get too low, deficiency symptoms may occur. A deficiency should be discussed with a physician, who can recommend dietary changes or supplements when necessary.

BONE LOSS

A low level of calcium, which is called hypocalcemia, is difficult to diagnose because in the early stages, there are often no symptoms, says the Office of Dietary Supplements. However, without enough calcium, the bones can become frail and susceptible to fractures. If left untreated, osteoporosis can develop. In some cases, a fracture is the only warning sign of weak bones. Since a calcium deficiency, bone loss and osteoporosis can all exist without causing symptoms, women should get regular bone-density tests starting around age 40, unless there are risk factors present. In addition, during routine physical exams, blood tests that can detect calcium levels should be done.

Numbness and Muscle Spasms

If a calcium deficiency continues untreated, it can affect the ability of the nerves to send signals properly. This can lead to generalized numbness and tingling sensations, especially in the fingers, toes and face, says the Cleveland Clinic. Some patients may even experience muscle spasms or paralysis in those areas. Uncontrollable movements that mimic Parkinson's disease can also occur. Over time, the muscles may become stiff and painful.

Irregular Heart Rhythms

Calcium deficiencies can occur due to thyroid disease, kidney disease, intestinal disorders that inhibit the digestion of calcium or vitamin D, alcoholism and a diet low in calcium and vitamin D. **In severe deficiencies, low levels of calcium can cause irregular heart rhythms and palpitations**, which may or may not be accompanied by fainting or dizzy spells, says the American Academy of Family Physicians. Also, blood pressure readings can go either too high or too low. Some patients may even experience difficulty breathing or shortness of breath.

Seizures and Coma

The brain also requires calcium to function properly, and if a deficiency occurs confusion, fatigue and psychosis may develop. Hypocalcemia can be fatal, and patients may go into seizures, convulsions or a coma unless proper medical attention is received. In these cases, a patient would need to be hospitalized and receive calcium intravenously.

Arthritic Pain

One thing I forgot to tell anyone suffering from arthritic pain is that an additional therapy of taking SOD (super oxide dismutase) –a natural antioxidant that is found in your body, has been shown to dramatically reduce the pain of crippling arthritis. LEF published a little news blurb stating that a number of people who had to use a cane due to arthritic pain were able to throw their canes away after 2 weeks of taking SODzyme which you can get from , of course, Life Extension Foundation. I know it worked in one of my friends who was scheduled to get knee replacement surgery. I put him on 400mg of SODzyme and a small amount of Vitamin D3 and within a month he got rid of his cane and was bouncing up and down the stairs with no problem. His knee replacement surgeon just had to reschedule and wait. It also worked in an old arthritic dog I had at the time.

Another Mystery Solved

Many years ago I had heard that skim milk causes prostate cancer some how. That just never made sense to me and stuck in my craw since I loved skim milk and still drank it since I did not believe the study. It turns out after reading the book about Vitamin K2 and the Calcium paradox. By Dr. Kate Bleau, I realized the study was correct, but they had it backwards. Prostate cancer is not caused by skim milk, it is prevented by ingesting milk fat! Why? Milk fat has Vitamin K2 in it which prevents prostate cancer.

This solves another mystery. You may read on various websites such as Dr. Mercola's (excellent site) that too high Vitamin D3 levels cause prostate cancer. Now we know why. Very high D3 levels without K2 supplementation depletes your K2, and the K2 depletion is what seems to cause prostate cancer. AHHHH I love it when all the weird puzzle pieces fit together!

20.
Longevity and Vitamin D3

A reader from Scotland just sent me an interesting article that got my mind churning again. The article says there was a study done of people who reached age 90 or more and their relatives and it turned out that those that lived the longest tended to have a significantly LOWER level of D3 in their blood!! The study examined 380 Dutch families with members who lived into their 90's that they found in the Leiden Longevity study. And to their surprise they found that naturally low levels of vitamin D may go hand-in-hand with a genetic resistance to ageing!

What the hell? Was my first reaction. But these weird puzzle pieces always seem to tell you something important. It then dawned on me that this study was likely done on people from a northern climate. And it also likely did not control for one important variable-the ability to tan and not burn in the sun. I am guessing that all the long livers that had low D3 levels are at the cutting edge of human evolution when it comes to the Vitamin D3 deficiency/illness connection.

So it then kind of jumped out at me. There is nothing inherently good for you about Vitamin D3, all it is a piece of information your body uses to turn on and off genes in reaction to information about your environment regarding the sun and what season it is. As humans move from sunnier to colder darker latitudes, the first settlers will become afflicted with the many diseases caused by lack of sun/lack of D3.

Many will die and not pass on their genes. The survivors will have evolved ways to make more D3 with less sun, and eventually over time might lose the need for D3 completely. How could they do this? Just by evolving some sort of mechanism that stimulates their Vitamin D3 receptors without the need for Vitamin D3 or sun. This evolution is likely going on in us humans, and these low D3 long-livers are getting past the need for D3 to thrive. They are probably the really pale people that cannot tan at all and always try to stay out of the sun. This then begs an interesting question: Does your ability to "not burn" (or tan) in the sun mark the degree to which Vitamin D3 supplementation will benefit you in preventing and treating diseases? Also, this study should not be interpreted to mean that D3 is bad for you, it might even turn out that had these long-livers boosted their D3 levels they might have lived even longer.

Are there any animals that do not need D3? I have learned of one, the naked mole rat who lives 100% underground, and is about the size of a regular rat but can live up to 8 years with no D3 at all while the above ground rat only live up to three years in general. So maybe someday northern-living humans will evolve, like naked mole rats, into long-living albinos that need neither sunlight nor Vitamin D3 for their health.

Vitamin D and Magnesium

It is very interesting that just a few people who have contacted me said the Vitamin D3 did not make them feel so good, but when they added magnesium to their program, everything was working as expected. So if you aren't getting the results you expect, maybe try adding some magnesium. I looked it up and it turns out that high doses of Vitamin D3 can induce not only a Vitamin K2 deficiency, but also a magnesium deficiency.

Later Note- WARNING! A very few people who take high dose D3 complain of heart racing, large changes in blood pressure, kind of like the guy you just read about complaining about the mk7 form of K2. It turns out that for most of these people I have corresponded with-when they added large doses of magnesium for a few days and then dropped to a maintenance dose-all these symptoms went away. Your doctor will not likely test you for or know about a magnesium deficiency but as it turns out-most of the population is magnesium deficient. And one of the dangerous symptoms will be heart irregularities and your doctor might order up 10's of thousands of dollars of unnecessary tests and procedures when all you really needed was extra magnesium!

Ace your next Blood Sugar Exam

An astounding blood sugar secret has emerged that'll have folks lining up to see their doctors and looking forward to their lab results...

Because there's finally an easier way to give yourself an advantage when it comes to your blood sugar health -- so you can feel great, energized and confident to face whatever tests your doctor throws your way.

Discover how this incredible blood sugar secret could work for you...

Imagine that just as your life is ending, you're given a bonus: two more years.

What would you do with those 730 extra days? Travel? Do volunteer work? Spend more time with your kids or grandkids?

While you're pondering that, also ponder this: Dr. W.B. Grant of the Sunlight, Nutrition and Health Research Center in California believes it can be done.

Dr. Grant crunched some numbers and came up with this simple equation: Double your blood level of vitamin D and you'll have a very good shot at a longer life -- approximately two years, on average.

This assumes that your vitamin D level is already low (around 54 nanomoles per liter (or 22 ng/ml). But as we've seen with several studies, just about everyone has low D levels, unless you happen to live near the equator.

For his study, Dr. Grant looked at research regarding diseases that are known to drop in risk when D levels are high. He determined that a D level of around 110 nanomoles per liter (44 ng/ml) would reduce risk of cancer, heart disease, infections, respiratory conditions and other diseases by 20 percent.

On average, that equals a gift of two extra years.

21.
Endnotes

[Here is the abstract of the new NIH paper and what the "professional" scientists are saying about it-Note Wang does not say that LH causes AD in his abstract but that GNRH agonists can treat neurodegeneration-one way it does this (I say the main way) is by suppressing LH-first mentioned anywhere in press or in private in my 1998 paper!]

"This is a very well referenced and comprehensive review of the literature and data surrounding the concepts of elevated **GNRH/LH** contributing to AD.

Probably most important, it was conducted and prepared by one of the leading neuroscientists at the NIH. Completely independent and with no ties to any private company."

Gonadotropin-releasing hormone receptor system: modulatoryrole in aging and neurodegeneration

Liyun Wang1, Wayne Chadwick1, Soo-Sung Park1, Yu Zhou1, Nathan Silver1, Bronwen

Martin2, and Stuart Maudsley1,*

1Receptor Pharmacology Unit, National Institute on Aging, National Institutes of Health, Biomedical

Research Center, 251 Bayview Boulevard, Baltimore MD 21224

2Metabolism Unit, Laboratory of Clinical Investigation, National Institute on Aging, National Institutes of Health, Biomedical Research Center, 251 Bayview Boulevard, Baltimore MD 21224

Abstract

Receptors for hormones of the hypothalamic-pituitary-gonadal axis are expressed throughout the brain. Age-related decline in gonadal reproductive hormones cause imbalances of this axis and many hormones in this axis have been functionally linked to neurodegenerative pathophysiology. Gonadotropin-releasing hormone (GnRH) plays a vital role in both central and peripheral reproductive regulation. GnRH has historically been known as a pituitary hormone; however, in the past few years, interest has been raised in GnRH actions at non-pituitary peripheral targets. GnRH ligands and receptors are found throughout the brain where they may act to control multiple higher functions such as learning and memory function and feeding behavior. The actions of GnRH in mammals are mediated by the activation of a unique rhodopsin-like G protein-coupled receptor that does not possess a cytoplasmic carboxyl terminal sequence. Activation of this receptor appears to mediate a wide variety of signaling mechanisms that show diversity in different tissues. Epidemiological support for a role of GnRH in central functions is evidenced by a reduction in neurodegenerative disease after GnRH agonist therapy. It has previously been considered that these effects were not via direct GnRH action in the brain, however recent data has pointed to a direct central action of these ligands outside the pituitary. We have therefore summarized the evidence supporting a central direct role of GnRH ligands and receptors in controlling central nervous physiology and pathophysiology. [and what follows is a reply by one of the scientists discussing the article]

Reply 3: NIH News!!! New paper suggests elevated LH behind AD

Prodiver replied 4 months, 1 week ago

Leuprolide acetate is the compound under study in the Phase II B trials. It is formulated in a patented biopolymer implant, developed by DURECT Corporation. According to the company, it uniquely releases a proprietary dosage level which is much higher than is used in previous applications of the compound to treat prostate cancer, endomitriosis or precocious puberty. LA has been shown to be very ...

note

My belief is that all the experiments that have been needed to be done to figure out any disease have already been performed! all one has to do is to manipulate the pub med database properly to figure out the answer to almost any question...here is what you get for "d3 deficiency causes osteoporosis"...a pathetic 79 results! and no titles that confirm the hypothesis-and just these meager 79 hits from all the research on osteoporosis and d3 from 1967 done to date!

Results: 79

Annual high-dose vitamin D3 and mental well-being: randomised controlled trial.

Sanders KM, Stuart AL, Williamson EJ, Jacka FN, Dodd S, Nicholson G, Berk M.Br J Psychiatry. 2011 May;198(5):357-64.

[Atypical celiac disease in a patient with type 1 diabetes mellitus and Hashimoto's thyreoiditis]. Schreiber FS, Ziob T, Vieth M, Elsbernd H.Dtsch Med Wochenschr. 2011 Jan;136(3):82-5. Epub 2011 Jan 11. German.

Cancer prevalence in osteoporotic women with low serum vitamin D levels.Veldhuis S, Wolbers F, Brouckaert O, Vermes I, Franke HR.Menopause. 2011 Mar;18(3):319-

Loss of bone mineral density in renal transplantation recipients.Unal A, Kocyigit I, Sipahioglu MH, Tokgoz B, Kavuncuoglu F, Oymak O, Utas C.Transplant Proc. 2010 Nov;42(9):3550-3.

[Vitamin D--an old vitamin in a new perspective].Gröber U. Med Monatsschr Pharm. 2010 Oct;33(10):376-83. Review. German.

Nursing home fractures: a challenge and a solution.Edlich RF, Mason SS, Swainston EM, Dahlstrom JJ, Gubler K, Long WB 3rd. J Environ Pathol Toxicol Oncol. 2010;29(1):7-11.

Critical reappraisal of vitamin D deficiency.Audran M, Briot K.Joint Bone Spine. 2010 Mar;77(2):115-9. Epub 2010 Jan 25. Review.

Vitamin D status and optimal supplementation in institutionalized adults with intellectual disability.Kilpinen-Loisa P, Arvio M, Ilvesmäki V, Mäkitie O.J Intellect Disabil Res. 2009 Dec;53(12):1014-23. Epub .

The effect of intramuscular vitamin D (cholecalciferol) on serum 25OH vitamin D levels in older female acute hospital admissions.

Nugent C, Roche K, Wilson S, Fitzgibbon M, Griffin D, Nichaidhin N, Mulkerrin E.Ir J Med Sci. 2010 Mar;179(1):57-61. Epub 2009 Aug 28.

The relation between osteoporosis and vitamin D levels and disease activity in ankylosing spondylitis.Mermerci Başkan B, Pekin Doğan Y, Sivas F, Bodur H, Ozoran K.Rheumatol Int. 2010 Jan;30(3):375-81. Epub 2009 Aug 14.

The relationship among renal injury, changed activity of renal 1-alpha hydroxylase and bone loss in elderly rats with insulin resistance or Type 2 diabetes mellitus.Huang CQ, Ma GZ, Tao MD, Ma XL, Liu QX, Feng J.J Endocrinol Invest.

Screening for celiac disease in patients with osteoporosis.Legroux-Gérot I, Leloire O, Blanckaert F, Tonnel F, Grardel B, Ducrocq JL, Cortet B.Joint Bone Spine. 2009 Mar;76(2):162-5. Epub 2009 Jan 29.

Dietary calcium and vitamin D2 supplementation with enhanced Lentinula edodes improves osteoporosis-like symptoms and induces duodenal and renal active calcium transport gene expression in mice.Lee GS, Byun HS, Yoon KH, Lee JS, Choi KC, Jeung EB.Eur J Nutr. 2009 Mar;48(2):75-83. Epub 2008 Dec

Changes in mineral metabolism in stage 3, 4, and 5 chronic kidney disease (not on dialysis)].Lorenzo Sellares V, Torregrosa V.Nefrologia. 2008;28 Suppl 3:67-

Vitamin D: a rapid review.Moyad MA. Urol Nurs. 2008 Oct;28(5):343-9, 384; quiz 350.

[Adequate level of vitamin D is essential for maintaining good health].Tukaj C.Postepy Hig Med Dosw (Online). 2008 Oct 9;62:502-10. Review. Polish.

Evaluation and correction of low vitamin D status.Binkley N, Krueger D.Curr Osteoporos Rep. 2008 Sep;6(3):95-9. Review.

Vitamin D therapy.Geller JL, Adams JS.Curr Osteoporos Rep. 2008 Mar;6(1):5-11. Review.

Vitamin D deficiency: a worldwide problem with health consequences.Holick MF, Chen TC.Am J Clin Nutr. 2008 Apr;87(4):1080S-6S. Review.

Sunlight, UV-radiation, vitamin D and skin cancer: how much sunlight do we need?Holick MF.Adv Exp Med Biol. 2008;624:1-15. Review.

Vitamin D therapy in clinical practice. One dose does not fit all.Ryan PJ.Int J Clin Pract. 2007 Nov;61(11):1894-9.

[Metabolic bone diseases].Jakob F.Internist (Berl). 2007 Oct;48 (10):1101-17. German.

Experimental osteoporosis induced by ovariectomy and vitamin D deficiency does not markedly affect fracture healing in rats.Melhus G, Solberg LB, Dimmen S, Madsen JE, Nordsletten L, Reinholt FP.Acta Orthop. 2007 Jun;78(3): 393-403.

[Vitamin D forming effectiveness of ultraviolet radiation from sunlight in different months in Budapest, Hungary].Bakos J, Mikó P.Orv Hetil. 2007 Feb 18;148(7):319-25. Hungarian.

The effect of cholecalciferol (vitamin D3) on the risk of fall and fracture: a meta-analysis.Jackson C, Gaugris S, Sen SS, Hosking D.QJM. 2007 Apr;100(4):185-92. Epub 2007 Feb 17. Review.

Vitamin D deficiency in residents of academic long-term care facilities despite having been prescribed vitamin D.Hamid Z, Riggs A, Spencer T, Redman C, Bodenner D.J Am Med Dir Assoc. 2007 Feb;8(2):71-5. Epub 2006 Oct 27.

Vitamin D status in patients with osteopenia or osteoporosis-- an audit of an endocrine clinic.Kocjan T, Tan TM, Conway GS, Prelevic G.Int J Vitam Nutr Res. 2006 Sep;76(5):307-13.

The effect of outfitting style on bone mineral density.Güler T, Sivas F, Başkan BM, Günesen O, Alemdaroğlu E, Ozoran K.Rheumatol Int. 2007 Jun;27(8):723-7. Epub 2007 Jan 16.

Duodenal calcium absorption in dexamethasone-treated mice: functional and molecular aspects.Van Cromphaut SJ, Stockmans I, Torrekens S, Van Herck E, Carmeliet G, Bouillon R.Arch Biochem Biophys. 2007 Apr 15;460(2):300-5. Epub 2006 Dec 12.

Vitamin D deficiency: A global perspective.Bandeira F, Griz L, Dreyer P, Eufrazino C, Bandeira C, Freese E.Arq Bras Endocrinol Metabol. 2006 Aug;50(4):640-6.

The problem of low levels of vitamin D and osteoporosis: use of combination therapy with alendronic acid and colecalciferol (vitamin D3).Epstein S. Drugs Aging. 2006;23(8):617-25.

The role of vitamin D for bone health and fracture prevention.Holick MF.Curr Osteoporos Rep. 2006 Sep;4(3):96-102. Review.

[Role of estrogen in aging and aging-related diseases].Inoue S.Seikagaku. 2006 Mar;78(3):257-61. Review. Japanese. No abstract available.

Vitamin D physiology.Lips P.Prog Biophys Mol Biol. 2006 Sep;92(1):4-8. Epub 2006 Feb 28.

NFkappaB decoy oligodeoxynucleotides ameliorates osteoporosis through inhibition of activation and differentiation of osteoclasts.Shimizu H, Nakagami H, Tsukamoto I, Morita S, Kunugiza Y, Tomita T, Yoshikawa H, Kaneda Y, Ogihara T, Morishita R.Gene Ther. 2006 Jun;13(12):933-41. Epub 2006 Mar 2.

Association of 1.25 vitamin D3 deficiency, disease activity and low bone mass in ankylosing spondylitis.Lange U, Teichmann J, Strunk J, Müller-Ladner U, Schmidt KL.Osteoporos Int. 2005 Dec;16(12):1999-2004. Epub 2005 Sep 20.

Peripheral genotype-phenotype correlations in Asian Indians with type 2 diabetes mellitus.Rao PV, Lu X, Pattee P, Turner M, Nandgaonkar S, Paturi BT, Roberts CT Jr, Nagalla SR.J Assoc Physicians India. 2005 Jun;53:521-6.

[Effect of combination treatment with estrogen and vitamin D3 on postmenopausal boneless].Mizunuma H.Clin Calcium. 2002 Jul;12(7):944-8. Japanese.

[Vitamin D deficiency as one of the causes of bone changes in chronic pancreatitis].Payer J, Killinger Z, Aleryany S, Kratochvíl'ová M, Ondrejka P.Vnitr Lek. 1999 May;45(5):281-3. Slovak.

[A pilot study of vitamin D in psychogeriatric patients: 82% is (severely) deficient].

Veeninga AT, Wielders JP, Oosterink J.Tijdschr Gerontol Geriatr. 2004 Oct;35(5):203-6. Dutch. Erratum in: Tijdschr Gerontol Geriatr. 2005 Apr;36(1):42. Dosage error in article text.

Functional indices of vitamin D status and ramifications of vitamin D deficiency.Heaney RP.Am J Clin Nutr. 2004 Dec;80 (6 Suppl):1706S-9S. Review.

Sunlight and vitamin D for bone health and prevention of autoimmune diseases, cancers, and cardiovascular disease.Holick MF.Am J Clin Nutr. 2004 Dec;80(6 Suppl):1678S-88S. Review.

[Insufficient calcium and vitamin D3. Malnutrition as fracture risk factor].[No authors listed]

MMW Fortschr Med. 2003 Oct 9;145(41):49. German. No abstract available.

The frequency of vitamin D deficiency in adults with Crohn's disease.Siffledeen JS, Siminoski K, Steinhart H, Greenberg G, Fedorak RN.Can J Gastroenterol. 2003 Aug;17(8):473-8.

Predominant factors associated with bone loss in liver transplant patients - after prolonged post-transplantation period.Segal E, Baruch Y, Kramsky R, Raz B, Tamir A, Ish-Shalom S.Clin Transplant. 2003 Feb;17(1):13-9.

Vitamin D3 metabolism in dogs.Hazewinkel HA, Tryfonidou MA.Mol Cell Endocrinol. 2002 Nov 29;197(1-2):23-33.

Hepatic osteodystrophy in chronic cholestasis: evidence for a multifactorial etiology.Klein GL, Soriano H, Shulman RJ, Levy M, Jones G, Langman CB.Pediatr Transplant. 2002 Apr;6(2):136-40.

Vitamin D status, parathyroid hormone and bone mineral density in patients with inflammatory bowel disease.Jahnsen J, Falch JA, Mowinckel P, Aadland Scand J Gastroenterol. 2002 Feb;37(2):192-9.

Vitamin D deficiency and secondary hyperparathyroidism in the elderly: consequences for bone loss and fractures and therapeutic implications.Lips P.Endocr Rev. 2001 Aug;22(4):477-501. Review.

1alpha-hydroxyvitamin D2 is less toxic but not bone selective relative to 1alpha-hydroxyvitamin D3 in ovariectomized rats.Weber K, Goldberg M, Stangassinger M, Erben RG.J Bone Miner Res. 2001 Apr;16(4):639-51.

Low vitamin D levels in outpatient postmenopausal women from a rheumatology clinic in Madrid, Spain: their relationship with bone mineral density.Aguado P, del Campo MT, Garcés MV, González-Casaús ML,

Bernad M, Gijón-Baños J, Martín Mola E, Torrijos A, Martínez ME.Osteoporos Int. 2000;11(9):739-44.

[Vitamin D deficiency in hospitalized patients].Killinger Z, Payer J Jr, Sládeková K, Kratochví'lová M, Ondrejka P.Vnitr Lek. 1999 Aug;45(8):473-5. Slovak.

A multidisciplinary renal clinic for corticosteroid-induced bone disease.Joy MS, Neyhart CD, Dooley MA.Pharmacotherapy. 2000 Feb;20(2):206-16.

Relative and combined effects of ethanol and protein deficiency on bone histology and mineral metabolism.Molina-Perez M, Gonzalez-Reimers E, Santolaria-Fernandez F, Martinez-Riera A, Rodriguez-Moreno F, Rodriguez-Rodriguez E, Milena-Abril A, Velasco-Vazquez J.Alcohol. 2000 Jan;20(1):1-8.

Abnormal bone and calcium metabolism in patients after stroke.Sato Y.Arch Phys Med Rehabil. 2000 Jan;81(1):117-21. Review.

1,25-Dihydroxyvitamin D3 in the pathogenesis and treatment of osteoporosis.DeLuca HF.Osteoporos Int. 1997;7 Suppl 3:S24-9. No abstract available.

The effect of season and latitude on in vitro vitamin D formation by sunlight in South Africa.Pettifor JM, Moodley GP, Hough FS, Koch H, Chen T, Lu Z, Holick MF.S Afr Med J. 1996 Oct;86(10):1270-2.

Vitamin D and bone health.holick MF.J Nutr. 1996 Apr;126(4 Suppl):1159S-64S. Review.

[Involutional osteoporosis--etiopathogenesis and treatment].Skalska A, Kocemba J.Folia Med Cracov. 1996;37(1-2):15-28. Review. Polish.

[Secondary hyperparathyroidism and tertiary hyperparathyroidism chronic renal failure, uremia].Morio K, Koide K.Nippon Rinsho. 1995 Apr;53(4):958-64. Review. Japanese.

[Therapeutic concepts in the treatment of postmenopausal osteoporosis].Leidig-Bruckner G, Ziegler R.Ther Umsch. 1994 Nov;51(11):737-47. German.

[Clinical applications expected in the future--osteoporosis].Fujita T.Nippon Rinsho. 1993 Apr;51(4):1004-10. Review. Japanese.

Vitamin D in bone formation.Seino Y, Ishizuka S, Shima M, Tanaka H.Osteoporos Int. 1993;3 Suppl 1:196-8. No abstract available.

Osteocalcin and its message: relationship to bone histology in magnesium-deprived rats.Carpenter TO, Mackowiak SJ, Troiano N, Gundberg CM.Am J Physiol. 1992 Jul;263(1 Pt 1):E107-14.

Different forms of alkaline phosphatase in adult rat femur. Effect of a vitamin D3-deficient diet and of a sorbitol-enriched diet.Tardivel S, Banide H, Porembska Z, Aymard P, Dupuis Y, Lacour B.Calcif Tissue Int. 1992 May;50(5):433-8.

Is there a role for vitamin D in osteoporosis?Lamberg-Allardt C.Calcif Tissue Int. 1991;49 Suppl:S46-9. Review.

Effects of vitamin D2 analogs on calcium metabolism in vitamin D-deficient rats and in MC3T3-E1 osteoblastic cells.Sato F, Ouchi Y, Okamoto Y, Kaneki M, Nakamura T, Ikekawa N, Orimo H.Res Exp Med (Berl). 1991;191(4):235-42.

Proliferation of tartrate-resistant acid phosphatase positive multinucleate cells in ovariectomized animals.Kalu DN.Proc Soc Exp Biol Med. 1990 Oct;195(1):70-4.

Studies of osteoporosis in Japan.Fujita T.Metabolism. 1990 Apr;39(4 Suppl 1):39-42.

Cytokines and osteoporosis.Fujita T, Matsui T, Nakao Y, Shiozawa S, Imai Y.Ann N Y Acad Sci. 1990;587:371-5. Review.

Abnormalities in parathyroid hormone secretion and 1,25-dihydroxyvitamin D3 formation in women with osteoporosis.Franz KB.N Engl J Med. 1989 Jun 22;320(25):1697-8. No abstract available.

Reversible bone loss in women treated with GnRH-agonists for endometriosis and uterine leiomyoma.Waibel-Treber S, Minne HW, Scharla SH, Bremen T, Ziegler R, Leyendecker G.Hum Reprod. 1989 May;4(4):384-8.

[Osteoporosis as a cause of pathologic fracture].Minne HW.Langenbecks Arch Chir Suppl II Verh Dtsch Ges Chir. 1989:493-502. Review. German.

Proximal femoral fractures.Hofeldt F.Clin Orthop Relat Res. 1987 May;(218):12-8. Review.

[Evaluation of the effects of anabolic steroids, calcitonin and 25-hydroxycholecalciferol on the spongy bone of rats].Carrozzo M, Cantatore FP, Pallante R, Lo Sasso F, D'Amore M, Pipitone V.Rev Rhum Mal Osteoartic. 1985 Jan;52(1):17-9. French.

1 alpha-Hydroxycholecalciferol and calcium deficiency osteoporosis in adult rats.Lindholm TS.Scand J Rheumatol. 1979;8(4):257-63.

Effect of vitamin D in fluoride-treated rats.Chapman SK, Malagodi MH, Thomas WC Jr.Clin Orthop Relat Res. 1978 Jan-Feb;(130):289-96.

The effect of 1alpha-hydroxyvitamin D3 with and without oestrogens on calcium balance in post-menopausal women.Marshall DH, Nordin BE.Clin Endocrinol (Oxf). 1977 Dec;7 Suppl:159s-168s.

Postmenopausal osteoporosis: the effect of parathormone and large dose vitamin D3 on the serum calcium level in sex hormone deficient rats.Holló I, Boross M, Steczek K, Szücs J.Acta Med Acad Sci Hung. 1975;32(3-4):255-9.

An Article:

THE STRANGE, DISTRESSING HISTORY AND FANTASTIC PROMISE OF HIGH-DOSE VITAMIN D

About 4,600 million years ago our solar system was formed when a huge cloud of dust leftover from an exploding star started collapsing. At first a large ball started to form in the center of the spiraling mass. Over time it contracted and coalesced into a perfect sphere...It was such a big ball that as gravity pulled all the matter together tighter and tighter , the dust and debris condensed so much that the ball caught on fire and started spitting out light and heat and cosmic rays of all kinds including ultraviolet (UV). Thus, with the birth of our sun came visible light and invisible ultraviolet light.

The newly burning sun was surrounded by rings of matter which over time collided this way and that until a number of smaller globes formed which are today's planets. There was not enough gravity or enough dust for these smaller bodies to catch fire and become stars, so most became cold solid spheres with just enough gravity to give them heated molten cores. One of these planets was the Earth, another was called Theia.

And the ball of matter called earth started rapidly spinning while at the same time slowly following a circular annual path around the sun. Initially everything was perfect, the earth spun on its axis perfectly vertical, upright like a top, while it traveled around the sun every year in a perfect circle.

Because the earth stood straight up and down as it traveled around the sun, there were no seasons anywhere. Everywhere on the earth each day was just as long as each night no matter where one was on the earth. At the equator or at the poles it made no difference. The only thing that varied was the intensity of the sunlight as the poles were further away from the sun than the equator. But the length of the day and the length of the night, everywhere on earth, were equal. If this situation occurred with our 24 hour day today, the sun would shine for 12 hours, and then the night would last for 12 hours everywhere on the earth, even at the poles, all the time forever.

But this perfect state of affairs was not to last.

And there are a number of reasonable different explanations for what happened next, any of which could be true, but for our purposes, the following scenario most conveniently allows us to continue our history.

Somewhere amongst the other planets lurked a rogue eccentric about the size of Mars named Theia, for the Greek Goddess who was the mother of the Moon goddess Selene. Unlike other planets, Theia was made mostly of iron.

For some reason Theia did not obey the rules of properly orbiting the sun in a perfect circle, but instead was almost violently erratic, threatening all the other perfect planets with a possible collision.

And then one day it happened…Theia's and Earth's orbits intersected in both time and place, and a collision of planets the magnitude of which had never before been seen nor ever would be seen again took place. It must have been a horrible sight to see!

A slow motion train wreck of the two infinitely huge fiery Gods might have been a good way to describe it...Like something one might read about in the Hindu scriptures. Like an ant of an ant of an ant.....watching two giant elephants fight in the sky. Most of Theia's mass became the molten iron core of the earth that generates a magnetic shield that protects us from cosmic rays and by creating conditions for the ozone layer to exist also protects us from excessive UV rays.

Theia came in from its skewed erratic path... and hit the earth at an angle different to earth's orbit. The two planets exploded in slow motion...exploding into one giant glowing melting fireball of lava, and the force was such that material enough for a small planet was ejected from the combined Earth & Theia. The amount of matter ejected from the fireball was equivalent to about $1/50^{th}$ of the matter of the new bigger earth.

This huge ejected mass shot off from the earth like a fiery rocket, but at about 240,000 miles away from the exploding earth the debris was finally captured by this new, bigger earth's gravity. And thus the moon was born and instantly married to the earth but took many thousands of years to condense into a perfect sphere. Although the moon formed from $1/50^{th}$ the matter on the earth, it sported an impressively big diameter equal to $1/4^{th}$ that of the earth's.

Because the moon was created from ejected debris from the earth, the moon was formed from matter that was rotating at the same speed the earth was at the time of the collision. Thus to us on earth it appears that the moon does not rotate, and that may be why we only see one side of the moon facing the earth at all times while it circles around us-because the material that makes the moon originally came from our spinning earth.

Now, the important thing for our purposes is that the rogue planet Theia....slammed into the earth at an angle...at a steep enough angle as to tilt the earth's perfectly vertical axis down by about 24 degrees. From that day forward the earth's axis would no longer be perfectly vertical, but tilted at 24 degrees away from / and 24 degrees towards the sun –depending on the season. From that day forward the earth would have dramatic changes in seasons every year which would be more and more extreme the further away one went from the equator.

And with the creation of the moon, this tilt in the earth's axis was glued into place by the moon's gravity...To forever remain at 24 degrees, to remain with the earth as long as the moon- to forever give the earth dramatic seasons in the northern and southern latitudes.

The most dramatic change in seasons is to be found at the poles; instead of experiencing days and nights of equal length as before. After the collision, the earth's poles now, every year, experience 6 months of complete darkness followed by 6 months of 24 hour/day sun and will continue in this state as long as the moon orbits the earth.

Well sooner or later after the creation of the moon and the seasons, simple single cell life forms somehow arose on planet earth-maybe 4.2 billion years ago.

Now nobody knows for sure if a bunch of chemicals on earth just started to self-assemble to create life, or if replicating life forms came to earth on a comet.

What IS known is that all life forms share the same genetic code. Basically all life on earth shares a language written with an alphabet of just 4 letters G, C, A or T....So we know for sure, like Darwin said, we are all related to that original organism that was the first life form that is the beginning of the evolutionary tree of life.

Now for comparison, our computers' machine language consists of a language written with only two symbols in its alphabet...just 1's and 0's. This might give you an idea of how advanced evolution is regarding information management. Evolution is very clever and very patient.

So billions of years ago the earth became tilted at 24 degrees long before the dawn of life on earth... ...Now let us fast forward a billion years or so from after the Collision, and we would find the Earth's first simple life forms were evolving:

maybe near the equator, maybe not.

But regardless of where they originated, they spread, east, west, but more importantly north and south. They were just single cells.

What did these first life forms do for a living? Not much-all they did was turn sunlight into stored energy/sugars via photosynthesis, reproduce like crazy, and spread geographically. Later life forms would evolve to become multi-cellular organisms, to engage in predation, movement, hibernation, mating, migration, etc. But the important thing that all life forms did, beginning with single cell photosynthetic plants, was to evolve ways to cope with the earth's seasons.

What was important about earth's seasons? The overriding factor was that the further one moved away from the equator, the more extreme the seasons would become. The further away from the equator one moved, the longer and longer were the nights during the frozen winter.

Combining extreme changes in the length of day and night with the fact that the further north or south one traveled, the less the intensity of the sun, led to a situation where the earth was covered with terrible famine zones. These were zones where up to 6 months a year famines were created by the shutdown of photosynthesis which ultimately provides the food and energy for all of life. Also in these zones drops in temperature were so extreme that almost everything became frozen solid unless evolution created some sort of special protection against it.

From the very first days, all life decided on one signal, to let it know that it was summertime, a time of abundance, a time when life was easy, and the cotton was high. The signal also disappeared in the winter...to let life know that the danger of starvation, freezing, and death was very real and that total extinction was more likely than survival, that it was time to hunker down and wait it out. That signal was the ultraviolet light given off by the sun. Invisible to the animal eye, but very visible to their skin or fur. And that signal became weaker and weaker the further away life got from the equator....and became less and less as the nights got longer and the days shorter.

What does evolution want life to do in the winter famine zones? It wants life to stop moving, to conserve resources, conserve energy, conserve heat; it wants life to fatten up before the famine occurs. It wants life to switch to survival mode, to conserve all resources, and perform just enough metabolic processes and repairs for life to get by…it wants to change life's physiology to prevent freezing damage, to make repairs with as few resources as possible, and wait for the good times and resources to return.

So what was the final outcome of this tug of war between summer abundance and frozen winter famine? It was a signal that all life obeys, the signal of ultraviolet light. In all life forms, both plant and animal, fungus, and bacteria…whenever life is exposed to UV rays it produces a hormonal signal which we call Vitamin D. If the UV exposure lessens or gets weaker, Vitamin D levels drop. Vitamin D levels are basically a prediction tool that life's DNA uses to tell an organism how to prepare for the next few months. And the signal accumulates and is stored or dissipates and is released over time in life's fatty tissues, so the signal that an organism gets any particular day is determined by a moving average of the UV exposure it has received over the last several months.

Well let's fast forward about 4 billion years or so.

Many of us humans living in the northern and southern latitudes have totally forgotten about this law of the earth. With our white skin, with our grocery stores full of summer foods all year round, with our heated and lighted houses, warm coats, and our 24/7 life styles, we wandering humans have just plain forgotten about the dangers of the death and extinction zones we live in. But just look outside next time you walk down a winter street. The trees haven't forgotten…they shut down completely and freeze solid, losing all their leaves....waiting for the UV signals of spring to come back to life...The birds and squirrels haven't forgotten....You don't see them at all for most of the winter, and most head for more tropical climates...But we humans go about our business like nothing at all is happening....No longer obeying the universal danger signal of low levels of UV light.

But what about earlier....when apes were becoming humans?

Let's look at our apelike ancestors who eventually evolved into us, likely starting somewhere near the equator in Africa.

Long before the discovery of agriculture allowed large civilizations like ancient Egypt or the Mayans to form, humans and proto-humans are thought to have existed in small groups of hunter gatherers who might follow herds of animals to hunt and sustain themselves. Thousands to millions of these small groups likely often wandered huge distances to avoid famines and chase herds of animals. It is certain that they wandered both north and south and back again. This likely went on for hundreds of thousands if not millions of years. Most of these small groups, just like all the small groups of Neanderthals went completely extinct- nothing left of them but dust and the 3% of our human DNA that came from interbreeding with the Neanderthals.. Only a few twigs of a very few branches on the evolutionary tree survived and continued surviving successfully just enough to pass some of their genes into the future, into our modern human gene pool.

So how did these very few lucky groups manage to survive their wanderings on the planet? To survive repeated forays into famine zones where there was no food for up to 6 months at a time, to survive through instant ice ages, or volcanic winters where eruptions or meteorite strikes blotted out the sun from the sky for months at a time?

They must logically have evolved the ability to undergo some sort of hibernation when they encountered winter/famine like conditions. Maybe it wasn't the same as a bear's hibernating where a 70% drop in D3 levels in the fall triggers overeating and a weight gain of 70% preceding a 4 month sleep; but it might have been. But from what can be gleaned from the host of diseases that humans face as they move further and further away from the equator we can get somewhat of an idea of what ancient human hibernation entailed.

As the sun became weaker and weaker as groups moved north or south, it would provide a signal , a drop in the UV light which led to reduced Vitamin D3 production in the skin or on the fur, that winter was coming, a signal to overeat and put on as much weight as possible to get ready for the famine. Ravenous hunger would take over, and these early humans would eat everything in sight -everything tasted great, and if they found enough food, they got fat. As the sun got weaker and days shorter as the earth spun away from the sun, soon a great tiredness would overtake the pack. They would find a cave or shelter and hunker down. And those that did not want hunker down were inflicted with ailments that would limit their desire to move about or physical ability to move around: things like depression, the flu, arthritis, MS, asthma, irritable bowel syndrome, anything to keep individuals from wandering around in the famine and burning precious energy...When the sun got strong again and the UV signal was re-encountered....evolution decided to undo the damage it had inflicted during the winter for the human/apes' own good...Depression lifted, the flu went away, arthritis and MS magically resolved...Lungs grew back their capacity...

Recently, scientists have determined that human DNA consists of up to 3% of DNA that came from Neanderthals which are primitive hominoids that lived in Northern Europe for several 100,000 years before the human migration out of Africa. What is fascinating about the Neanderthal DNA is that the genes we carry from them are primarily involved with the development of our skin and hair. They also gave us genes that cause lupus and Crohn's Disease-both diseases that seem to be curable with high dose D3. Apparently Neanderthals probably gave northern humans their white skin and straight hair as it turns out that Sub Saharan Africans have no Neanderthal DNA.

Another adaptation that evolved in hominids was that low Vitamin D levels also told the body to increase its blood sugar and blood pressure to reduce the risk of the organs being damaged by freezing/crystallization of water turning the body's water into ice crystal daggers and puncturing cells and membranes and organelles throughout the body. Higher sugar levels in the blood reduced blood's freezing point and is a strategy employed by all sorts of animals that survive freezing in winter including amphibians, insects, and reptiles. In fact, antifreeze for cars is made of ethylene glycol, a sugar. Increased blood pressure also reduces the freezing temperature of water since water expands as it freezes into ice. Increased water pressure fights against the expansion/crystallization process. Today we see remnants of this survival adaptation and call it diabetes and high blood pressure or "metabolic syndrome" which is quite strongly associated with low vitamin d levels.

Groups that did not receive this hint from evolution to hunker down during winter surely starved to death and went extinct...and those who did not prepare their bodies to prevent freezing damage also suffered the same fate. The only survivors were those who reacted appropriately to the lack of sun and heat.......and waited out the season of freezing and starvation in the famine zone by conserving energy and changing their blood physiology towards a high pressure, sugary antifreeze.

Today we also see a snapshot of the evidence of this eternal process in the skin colors of various native peoples at different latitudes.

Groups that lived around the equator quickly evolved dark skin which filters out UV light and protects against sunburn caused by the intense UV rays. But this also filtered out a lot of the UV summer-is-here signal. Those groups that had migrated north or south and decided to stay there still needed their D3 signal to tell the body it was okay to initiate repairs, that resources were available, but the sun was too weak to give it. So they lost their dark skin color so the signal would not be interfered with by protective pigmenting. They became white and very sensitive to the sun. Just a little sun would give them the signal that winter and the famine was over. There was no longer a need for year round dark skin.

Those that remained at the equator which was basically devoid of seasons did not need the UV signal that the famine was over but needed protection from the much stronger UV rays to prevent sunburn. They remained black or became black if they had migrated back south form the north. People in between the north and the equator became brown...a nice compromise.

So our apelike ancestors and humans of even just a few hundred years ago went around living in this world of seasons controlled by invisible UV light, blissfully ignorant of UV's importance and its complete control and stranglehold on their lives and health.

For most of human history the negative effects of UV deficiency (winter) on us hominids was likely chalked up to "evil spirits".

But finally in the year 1650, we humans started to figure out what was going on. It was just a scratch on the surface of the entire story and science of UV and D3 ......but it was the first tiny glimpse into the mystery.

It was the 17th century when the increasing urbanization in England and the rampant burning of coal blocked out the sun and began to lead to widespread Vitamin D deficiencies in newborns and their mothers. It was enough to trigger widespread Vitamin D deficiencies in the newborns that were kept mostly indoors. This led to the observation by a British doctor of a new disease called rickets that had never been seen before. Rickets led to many skeletal deformities in children aged 6 months to 2 years old. But once the children started playing outdoors after age 2, the disease seemed to go into remission.[1] Also around this time, another doctor described the problems of delivering infants through women's rickety pelvises. A few centuries later, a German doctor, in 1824 discovered that cod-liver oil which had been used medicinally for a long time could be used to treat rickets.[2] And it wasn't until1906 that an English biochemist discovered vitamins as being dietary factors that were necessary to prevent diseases.

There was another line of research going on around this time stimulated by the discovery of mysterious rays emitted by the newly invented mercury vapor lamp in 1901. [3] This new kind of light gave off an ugly greenish glow but it was heavily loaded with ultraviolet rays. Later in the 1920's researchers in both the US and England found that these mysterious rays when shined on rats that had rickets, would cure them. But much to their surprise they found that removing the rats and irradiating their empty cages also cured the rats of rickets! [4] This initially set off a frenzy about the new curative mercury lamp rays which led to a booming new industry of miracle lamps. And if you look back at supposed "quack" devices that people used to cure disease in the 1920's you will find lots of devices that emitted UV rays. The funny thing is that now that we know what we know, these were not quack devices but devices that might have had some beneficial effects similar to taking Vitamin D3 or Cod Liver oil. You can see these antique miracle ray machines still for sale as quack medicine curiosities on e-bay.

Can you imagine being one of these scientists and finding that these mysterious UV rays not only cured rats of rickets when you exposed them to the rays..but also got rid of rickets when you irradiated JUST THEIR EMPTY CAGES! What magic it must have seemed!!

This then led scientists to think that somehow the rays altered the air in their cages to a curative nature.

This was then tested by having the assistants blow the air out of their cages before the rats were returned and lo and behold the rats got rickets! [5]

For a few years they thought UV radiation altered the air towards curative powers and pushed the scientific community towards the idea that disease came from "bad air". And thus you found tuberculosis patients prescribed a therapy of sitting in large wooden structures situated out in the windy western plains with various holes in them to circulate good air around them, (called sanatoriums). Ironically it turns out that low D3 levels are now thought to be the primary cause of tuberculosis.

It was later found the assistant who had blown the air out of the rats' cages also removed all the sawdust bedding first so that it would not blow back in his face. A later experiment where the bedding was not disturbed when the air was blown out, found that irradiating empty rat cages with UV light and leaving the sawdust bedding and whatever it contained (i.e. feces and rat oil) in place led to rats being cured of their rickets! [6]

This drove the scientists crazy! But they finally got it right when they stacked rat cages on top of each other. They found that irradiated empty cages prevented rickets in the rats who lived in these cages and the ones who lived below, but not the ones who lived above! [7] With this they finally realized the curative substance was a substance with gravity. But this part of the history of Vitamin D3 discovery has been basically ignored, but I find it fascinating.

Finally, in 1922, scientists working with dogs kept indoors had all this information to work with when they finally discovered a dietary substance contained in cod liver oil could prevent rickets in dogs raised completely indoors and they called it Vitamin D because Vitamins A,B and C, had already been discovered....but I say the true discoverers were the relatively unknown scientists who did the rat cage experiments who discovered Vitamin D2!

It turns out that the scientists doing the dog experiments had discovered cod liver oil contains the animal form of Vitamin D-Vitamin D3, not the slightly different plant form of Vitamin D2.

While the dog experiments eventually led to the isolation of Vitamin D3, the commercialization of Vitamin D in the 1920's came from mass production of the plant form of Vitamin D-vitamin D2 which came from irradiating plant products with UV light. In 1923, American biochemist Harry Steenbock at the University of Wisconsin demonstrated that irradiation by ultraviolet light increased the vitamin D content of foods and other organic materials. It was Steenbock who discovered that after irradiating rodent food, that the rodents were cured of rickets. [8]

While most scientists of the day did not file patents on products of university research, Steenbock broke protocol and patented his irradiation technique to boost the Vitamin D2 content of foodstuffs, most memorably for milk. He then transferred his patent to the Wisconsin Alumni Research Fund (WARF) of the University of Wisconsin and for many years hundreds of millions flowed into the fund turning WARF into a research powerhouse whose inventions include the still popular blood thinner named WARFarin in honor of the fund. Finally in 1943, his patent was invalidated by a federal appeals court that stated Steenbock's process was a discovery and not an invention and was no more patentable than trying to patent the use of sunshine to boost Vitamin D levels in grass.

It turns out that irradiating many organic substances with UV rays cause Vitamin D to be created from a ubiquitous organic substrate. Vitamin D is created by irradiating milk or even mushrooms. Because the first form of Vitamin D known to man which was the plant form-Vitamin D2 which came from irradiating mushrooms, Vitamin D2 was given the name ergocalciferol which comes from the word ergot meaning fungus or mushroom. Vitamin D2 is the plant form of biologically active (in humans) of Vitamin D…and it turns out that it is from $1/4^{th}$ to $1/16$th as active as the animal form of Vitamin D which is known as Vitamin D3 or cholecalciferol which was isolated much later than the D2 version.

The active forms of Vitamin D (Vitamin D3 and Vitamin D2) are not really vitamins at all…They are actually very potent hormones. Vitamin D was just mislabeled as a vitamin when it was discovered in the 1920's because they mistakenly thought it only came from the diet. But Vitamin D3 can be made in animals by UV light hitting the skin or fur. What happens in animals is that the UV light catalyzes the conversion of a form of cholesterol (7-dehydrocholesterol) into Vitamin D3. In humans this occurs in or on the skin, while in animals it occurs on their fur and they ingest the Vitamin D3 during grooming.

Vitamin D3 is actually a hormone that provides information to the DNA in every cell in your body....to tell the DNA to do things or not to do things. It is estimated to control at least 1000 different genes either by turning them on or turning them off. It does this by attaching to very small receptors that are attached to genes in your DNA called VDR's=Vitamin D Receptors. But the trigger happy vitamin-naming scientists jumped the gun and classified the hormone Vitamin D3 as a Vitamin when it is not because they first discovered it in the diet. This mislabeling persists to this day and obscures the importance of this vital life-giving hormone.

Other than its role in helping your body absorb calcium, for the most part there is nothing inherently good or bad about Vitamin D, other than the information it provides to your DNA ...it is primarily a molecular form of information-just as most hormones are. But if you don't get this information, you will surely die!

So what is the vital information that Vitamin D2 or D3 gives to your DNA that is so important? As you already know, the hypothesis is that it tells your DNA that the sun is shining! Now that's as far as you had to go to then move in the direction of coming up with a pretty robust theory of the cause and cure for most human diseases. We will get into this in detail at the latter part of this article. But now let's get back to the strange history of Vitamin D, in particular Big Pharma's and the FDA's attempts to outlaw it.

After the discovery of a way to easily and cheaply make large amounts of Vitamin D2 by shining UV light on organic matter, the US public in the late 1920's started taking it in droves. Also dozens of foods were being fortified with vitamin D by irradiation including hot dogs and beer. Newspaper articles talked of the miracle of sunshine in a pill and touting its many health benefits. According to one scientist's account the average person in the late 1920's and early 1930's was taking 20mg of Vitamin D2 a day , and soon the hospitals were empty-nobody was getting sick anymore. The hospitals were all about to go bankrupt along with the doctors and drug companies.[9]

At about this time studies with much higher doses than the human equivalent of 20mg a day were being undertaken on dogs by various researchers. Some studies suggested toxicities were being encountered at doses higher than 20 mg per day but later it turned out that toxicity was thought to be mostly being caused by impurities in the preparation process and that later, better, methods produced virtually non- toxic Vitamin D2. (However, taking much higher levels than this, like ingesting almost any substance in very excessive amounts, can be dangerous and ultimately toxic-so one does need to be careful with experimentation).

So one version of events is that some in the drug/medical industry latched onto the idea of Vitamin D toxicity to try and get Vitamin D outlawed. Their first action was to change the unit of measurement of Vitamin D2 from milligrams to International Units which we use today. All of the sudden 20 mg became 1 million International Units...which sounds much scarier indeed! Also, a study was performed where 7 medical students were convinced to take massive enough doses of Vitamin D to kill a horse, and lo and behold the students got very sick, the experiment was stopped and they recovered. [10]That was all that was needed and medical authorities pressured Vitamin D manufacturers and retailers to take Vitamin D off the market.

As expected there was a public outcry and the government in 1928 decided to commission a comprehensive study of the question of Vitamin D toxicity with the University of Illinois at Chicago. The study lasted 9 years, involved hundreds of doctors and 773 humans and 63 dogs, and resulted in what is known as the Steck report (but often mistakenly called the Streck report on the internet) . [11] This report basically concluded that doses up to 20,000 IU per kilogram per day (or 1 million IU's per the typical woman of 50 kgs/110 pounds) were safely tolerated in dogs for indeterminate lengths of time even when taken for years. The report blamed prior cases of toxicity on improper production techniques and stated that the new "Whittier" process eliminated Vitamin D toxicity. Amongst the humans, who were given does of up to 200,000 IU a day for periods of seven days to five years there were no deaths. And one of the authors of the report took 3 million IU's a day for 15 days without any evidence of disturbance of any kind. And finally they found vitamin D intoxication by taking much higher amounts of Vitamin D for short periods did not result in any recognizable permanent injury. The final conclusion was that the burden of proof had shifted to those who maintained the undesirability of high dose Vitamin D therapy.

Quite a few subsequent studies in the 30's and 40's showed that massive doses of Vitamin D2 were quite effective at treating and curing arthritis. [12]

(Now keep in mind they were using Vitamin D2 back then which is 1/4th to 1/16th as active as Vitamin D3. But translating this into a safe range of D3 we could infer a 100 pound person could safely ingest somewhere between 50,000 to 250,000 IU a day of D3. I would suggest not exceeding 50,000 IU a day for a 100 pounder until one gets their blood tested. AND to make sure one supplements with adequate amounts of Vitamin K2 which in my case was 1000 mcg per each 10,000 IU of D3 during my self-experiment to be described shortly.)

The American Medical Association and drug industry ignored these studies and the Steck report and continued to maintain that "Vitamin D in doses over 400 IU a day may be toxic"! And since the 1930's this has been the recommended amount of vitamin D we are all supposed to take according to doctors and the drug industry-just enough to keep us from getting rickets and our bones becoming soft!

To most outside observers, this behavior of the drug companies, doctors, and scientists, to knowingly declare something toxic that had so much promise for treating and curing diseases, with the intent of keeping people sick so they could make money, might seem unethical. There is an oath, invented by Hippocrates-the father of medicine- that supposedly all newly minted doctors take (98% in the US and only 50% in the UK) which includes the pledge.." I will prescribe regimens for the good of my patients according to my ability and my judgment and never do harm to anyone". I would think knowingly calling a healing substance "toxic" would be in violation of this pledge.

It might all sound so preposterous, like a huge evil conspiracy! But keep in mind this was in the 1930's at the same time the US Government and its US Department of

Health along with its doctors, scientists and researchers began the Tuskegee Syphilis project in 1932. This was a program where rural black men with syphilis were recruited into a program where they were told they would get free health care. The true object of the study was to just sit and watch and see what happened to humans with untreated syphilis. The study went on for 40 years until 1972!! And no one blew the whistle even when all the men could have been cured with penicillin when it started being mass produced in 1945. The US government just kept telling the study subjects they were getting medicine which was just placebo. So much for the suppression of Vitamin D being too evil for science, Big Pharma, and the US Government to get behind!

So scientists and drug companies were telling us in the 1930's that any amount of vitamin D over 400 IU's may be toxic.. But somehow the drug industry saw fit to create three new miracle drugs for use in treating cancer and other diseases with the brand names Dalsol, Deltalin, and Drisdol. Each of these drugs was nothing more than a daily pill containing 50,000 IU of vitamin D2 and a filler. The drug industry was not doing well during the depression years of the 1930's and these "new" drugs that actually worked saved them financially, all the while they were telling the public anything over 400 IU was toxic. (More than 400 IU being dangerous is especially ridiculous when you consider that whole body sunbathing for just thirty minutes produces 10,000 to 20,000 IU of Vitamin D3 in your skin!) [13]

Once the patent on Vitamin D was invalidated in 1943, the drug companies needed to somehow get Vitamin D back under their control. So, the campaign started in New York in 1944 when the attorney general Nathaniel Goldstein ruled that vitamins were drugs and could only be sold by pharmacists and registered drug stores. [14]This ruling was quickly challenged in court and overturned. But Big Pharma was not going to just give up easily.

In 1952 the FDA (Food & Drug Association) tried to outlaw the introduction of anything "new" into foods and consumables unless given advanced affirmative permission by the FDA. This power grab was rejected by the courts. In 1957 the FDA started prosecution of vendors of "malnutrition remedies" (AKA vitamins) and began using the term "quack".

In 1960 the FDA tried to limit the amount of folic acid in vitamins to .4 of a milligram even though years later this amount would be found to be too low and higher amounts were recommended for pregnant mothers to prevent neural tube defects in their newborns. In 1966 again the FDA tried to restrict access to vitamins by the food industry by proposing new controls on Vitamin D fortification. [15]

In 1973 the FDA banned the sale of higher dose Vitamin A and Vitamin D pills. This was later challenged by Linus Pauling, the Nobel Prize winning chemist, as a friend of the court in a lawsuit against the FDA.

In 1974 Congress reigned in the FDA's overreach and forced them to regulate vitamins as food and not drugs. In 1976 Congress also passed a bill blocking the FDA and the drug industry's attempts to block the sale of high dose vitamins. AND in 1977 the FDA dropped its plans to require a doctor's prescription for high dose vitamins.

But in 1979, the FDA tried again to get some vitamins classified as non-prescription drugs...another small first step towards later banning.

1992: The FDA with Texas state health inspectors raided vitamin retailers/ health food stores across the state and seized inventories and put people in jail accusing the businessmen of making false health claims about vitamins.

1993: FDA planned to regulate vitamins again and health claims about them.

Finally: in 1994 the people of the US had had enough and they forced Congress to pass the US Dietary Supplement Health and Education Act (DSHEA) which is basically "health-freedom" legislation. DSHEA defines supplements as foods, and puts the onus on the United States Food and Drug Administration (FDA) to prove that a supplement poses significant or unreasonable risk of harm rather than on the manufacturer to prove the supplement's safety, reversing the burden of evidence required of medicines.

They never quit though. In 2011 some corrupt, bought and paid for, nanny-statist US politicians tried a back door maneuver to regain control over vitamins and supplements by the FDA with their introduction of the Dietary Supplement Labeling Act of 2011.

Their intent was to overthrow the effect of the 1994 DSHEA law which led to consumers having wide access to dietary supplements. They wanted to change what was essentially a notification process into a costly approval process. The net effect of the proposed regulation was to reclassify many nutritional compounds currently on the market as new dietary ingredients requiring FDA approval. Luckily for the US population this recent backdoor power grab attempt also failed. But you can bet the corrupted, nanny-state politicians owned by Big Pharma will be at it again sooner or later-stay tuned.

And finally the CODEX attempted power grab which is ongoing right now:

The Codex Alimentarius Commission is an FAO/WHO United Nations entity whose purpose is to "create a set of international standards to guide the world's growing food industry and to protect the health of consumers."

Germany has been attempting to manipulate the Codex Committee on Nutrition and Foods for Special Dietary Use to further the interests of the German pharmaceutical industry, by raising regulatory standards so that only the big drug companies like Hoechst, Bayer, BASF, Degussa, Fresnius, Rhone-Poulenc, Sandoz, and Novo Nordisk can survive.

The German "Proposed Draft Guideline for Dietary Supplements" calls for the following:

-No dietary supplement can be sold for prophylactic (preventive or therapeutic) use; (goodbye Vitamin D!)

-No dietary supplement sold as a food can exceed potency (dosage) levels set by the commission; (goodbye high dose Vitamin D!)

-Codex standards for dietary supplements would become binding. (Government wins-you lose!)

-All new dietary supplements would automatically be banned unless they conform to Codex standards- which would require going through a very expensive drug-like approval process. (Wow! Are we going to put up with this??! Who do they think they are?)

If the US signs onto the Codex-the FDA will have the power to shut down health food stores and prohibit the sale of vitamins except by prescription only at approved drugstores.

To see what the future might hold for the sale of vitamins and supplements

all over the world under CODEX one needs only to go to Germany and try to stock up.. There are no competing brands placed out on accessible shelves. You can only get overpriced/undersized vitamins at special sterile stores called apothecaries which are staffed by pharmacists in clean white jackets. You are not allowed to freely touch the extremely overpriced vitamins which are kept safely behind the counter. The pharmacist will bring them to you and ask you many questions and ask to see your prescription.

In Germany there is a thing called "Die Rote List" where one can find a complete listing of international pharmaceutical firms that manufacture patented analogs of extremely overpriced dietary supplements sold as OTC and prescription drugs. Through this you can see who the companies are that are trying to manipulate the Codex process.

Now that we have the world's history of Vitamin D out of the way, let me now detail my own recent personal history with D.[16]

I have never been a person who easily accepted or even considered conspiracy theories. In fact my whole life I have been just the opposite- very dismissive of conspiracy theorists! But recently I am now starting to wonder. What is a possible conspiracy I might have uncovered?

The almost criminal advice that doctors have been giving us for years- To stay out of the sun, use sunscreen, and that too much Vitamin D is dangerous!!

When doctors started warning us in the 1980's to avoid the sun and use sunscreen, explosive increases in rates of obesity, autism, asthma, and other diseases have occurred! The First Lady of the United States-Michelle Obama is trying to fight obesity in kids by getting them to eat better and exercise more-but what if something else is causing their problems- like a lack of Vitamin D3 due to lack of sun?

As a child I had medical issues like asthma, ADHD, and scleroderma morphea. After age 28, I started accumulating injuries and issues that doctors could not easily heal such as yellow toenail fungus, a facial subcutaneous cyst, a hip-click, a bone spur on my elbow, a ganglion cyst on my wrist, and arthritic-popping shoulders and back.

After many years of independent research on aging and disease, I ran across an article about 8 years ago that suggested 80% of people with aches and pains are deficient in Vitamin D3 [17]. As soon as I read it I started taking 4,000 IU a day of Vitamin D3 (10X the daily recommended dose of 400 IU), and within a month almost all my arthritic issues went away. However, the hip click, yellow toenails, ganglion cyst, subcutaneous cyst, and hip click, stubbornly remained.

Flash forward about 6 years- my father, who had been taking 2000 IU of Vitamin D3 a day for years (5X the recommended daily dose) had his first Vitamin D3 blood test come back at 29 ng/ml..1 ng lower than the lowest end of the reference range-meaning he should already be dead! This was my Eureka moment! I guessed that my family might be genetically programmed to be low in D3, so I upped my dose to 20,000 IU a day, and later boosted it to 50,000 and even 100,000 IU a day- and the rest is (my) history.

Within a month I started feeling lots of energy and also pain in my bones and joints that had never healed properly. I was not scared because I had read that Vitamin D3 was considered the bone and joint remodeling hormone. I had also read that rats whose legs were broken and given D3 had perfectly healed breaks, while the control rats had breaks with a large callous remaining around the repair.

Within 5 months my yellow toenails were clearing up, my hip click was dissolving, my shoulders were being repaired even better than before (at 4,000 IU a day). And after a year, I noticed my bone spur on my elbow disappeared, my subcutaneous cyst popped and is gone, and my ganglion cyst shrank from the size of half a fleshy golf ball to that of a rock hard painless pea.

I wondered- why would evolution evolve a sunshine-activated hormone? This led me to the idea of the Incomplete Repair Syndrome where evolution thinks you are stuck in winter where resources will be scarce, so it will repair and maintain you just enough to get by and no more. Then, the D3 sunshine signal announces that summer is here and resources are available, your body will then undo the incomplete repairs and redo them properly using all the resources necessary.

I then found that a large drop in D3 levels, is a major signal for bears to prepare for hibernation which includes increasing body weight by 70%! [18] More research- and lo and behold , obese people are overwhelmingly deficient in Vitamin D3! This led me to the next idea of a higher level syndrome-the Human Hibernation Syndrome (HHS)- where if someone attains low levels of Vitamin D3 all year and all life-long by avoiding the sun and using sunscreen, they eventually will become obese to prepare for hibernation during the expected winter famine.

In addition to weight gain, HHS might also reduce the expenditure of precious energy. With this in mind, HHS might also promote depression to keep one house/cave-bound. Low D3 also makes humans more susceptible to the normally harmless flu, which requires a week in bed and further conserves precious energy. Arthritis? It discourages energy expenditure from running around, or it could just be part of the Incomplete Repair Syndrome- conserving precious calcium with incomplete repairs.

I then read or browsed all 52,000 science articles/studies from 1967 to present available on the Pub Med database for "Vitamin D" (now there are 55,000 articles!), and discovered that low D3 levels are associated with almost every disease known to man not caused by aging or genetic mutations.

Here is a small sample: autism, asthma, diabetes, severe hypoglycemia, chronic wounds, MS, lupus, kidney and lung diseases, 17 types of cancer, glaucoma, macular degeneration, Crohn's disease, IBS & UC, hypertension, rheumatoid arthritis, schizophrenia, allergies, tuberculosis, heart diseases, ulcers, cavities, Parkinson's, strokes, psoriasis , dandruff, all pregnancy complications, migraines, menstrual cramps, PMS, cavities and many more! Any common disease in humans seems to be caused by low levels of sun exposure and thus low levels of Vitamin D3 in your blood! It's quite easy to see which diseases are caused by low levels of Vitamin D3, you just need to look at the geographical distribution and incidence of the disease and if like most of them, they are much reduced at the equator and much higher in the extreme latitudes [19]...then it's clear –they are Vitamin D3 related and can be cured with high doses.

Now, if most diseases could be prevented by boosting your D3 from 30 ng/ml which is low but typical, to 80-100 ng/ml- or higher, what do you think would happen to the profits generated from Big Pharma's drugs, if it became known that D3 prevented and was the superior treatment for all these diseases? The profits and jobs would disappear overnight!

One might imagine a Dr. Evil-like, Big Pharma executive who somehow knows this information (and should know), thinking..."Vitamin D3 is the enemy of our existence! We must suppress the idea of taking high does D3 at all costs!!" Discovering the D3 deficiency disease link was not that hard of a nut for me to crack for me and for a lot of MDs with their books out there. And if we did it ,just little old us, how is it that all these billions and years of research by Big Pharma into all these different drugs, didn't find this out a long time ago!!??

Big Pharma's drugs all seem to be trying to mimic what high dose D3 does. But since their drugs are not D3, the sunshine hormone, their drugs have all sorts of nasty side effects.

Why would they feed us such dubious drugs if they have knowledge of the superior curative effects of high dose D3 (which they should)?

Answer: To make a profit-because they cannot patent Vitamin D3! They cannot patent sunshine!

So- I am beginning to wonder if there are a few Big Pharma execs who know this truth but decided to demonize D3 by creating a fear of scary side effects such as excess calcification of tissues (which can occur at doses of several million IU or more per day!-but probably only if you do not take ample Vitamin K2 with the D3) and drumming the idea into all med students that high dose D3 is very dangerous!

In my research on D3 I looked at all the science articles in Pub Med that describe Vitamin D3 toxicity and discovered almost all of them are reports of doctors' patients who took relatively huge doses of D3 for long periods and had no ill effects. The doctors were dumbfounded as it contradicted everything they had learned in med school!! (Side Note-One other thing I learned was that the effects of extreme high dose D3 are very similar to the effects of a Vitamin K2 deficiency-so if you try high dose D3 also take a lot of Vitamin K2.)[20]

So- am I now a paranoid believer in conspiracy theories like one where Big Pharma has intentionally taught doctors in med school that high dose D3 is bad for you so that they could go on selling their inferior, dangerous drugs to make huge profits? Not yet.

I would rather believe that this is all just a matter of some possible malfeasance by a small cabal of drug researchers back in the 1930's, and modern day incompetence along with Big Pharma's refusal to study high dose vitamin D3 because it cannot generate profits because it is not patentable.

As far as answering the question if today's drug companies and researchers actually know about the curative powers of high dose Vitamin D3 but are suppressing this knowledge for profit....I PUNT. I am almost scared to find the true answer!

So it is up to you to decide..

Is there something sinister behind the big pharma/medical community's exagerated fear of the dangers of high dose vitamin D3?

1. Claerr, Jennifer (February 6, 2008). "The History of Rickets, Scurvy and Other Nutritional Deficiencies". An Interesting Treatise on Human Stupidity. Yahoo! Voices. Archived from the original on 2013-03-26. Retrieved March 26, 2013. "URL references"

2. Schuette, D. Beobachtrugen Uber Den Nutzen Des Berger Leberthrans, Arch F. med. Erfahrung V2, 79, 1824.

3. "Peter Cooper Hewitt". Encyclopædia Britannica.

4. Forgotten Mysteries in the Early History of Vitamin D. Kenneth J. Carpenter1 and Ling Zhao. 1999 The American Society for Nutritional Sciences.

5. Ibid

6. Ibid

7. Ibid

8. SOLAR Ultraviolet Radiation AND Vitamin D A Historical Perspective Am J Public Health. 2007 October; 97(10): 1746–1754.

9. Quote attributed to the late famous Vitamin D/Calcium Researcher Dr. Carl Reich in Robert Bareoot's excellent book "The Disease Conspiracy-The FDA Suppression of Cures" 2006 page 141.

10. Ibid

11. Further Studies on Intoxication With Vitamin-D, was done by the University of Illinois, Chicago, Annuals of Internal Medicine, Volume 10, Number 7, January 1937,

12. Preliminary Report on Actiated Ergosterol (A form of high dose Vitamin-D in the treatment of chronic arthritis. G Snyder New York State journal of Medicine May 1940. And similar studies cited in Barefoot's book noted in #9 above.

13. Crissey SD, Ange KD, Jacobsen KL, Slifka KA, Bowen PE, Stacewicz-Sapuntzakis M, Langman CB, Sadler W, Kahn S (2003). "Serum concentrations of lipids, vitamin D metabolites, retinol, retinyl esters, tocopherols and selected carotenoids in twelve captive wild felid species at four zoos". The Journal of nutrition 133 (1): 160–6. PMID 12514284.

14. Vitamin Tablets Are Ruled Drugs And General Sale in State Curbed. New York Times, New York, NY: Jun 24, 1944 pg 1-2 pgs.

15. All these references can be found in Barefoot's book in #9.

16. Excerpts from my e-book: THE MIRACULOUS RESULTS OF EXTREMELY HIGH DOSES OF THE SUNSHINE HORMONE VITMIN D3 MY

EXPERIMENT WITH HUGE DOSES OF D3 FROM 25,000 to 50,000 to 100,000 IU A Day OVER A 1 YEAR PERIOD

17. Plotnikoff GA, Quigley JM. Prevalence of severe hypovitaminosis D in patients with persistent, nonspecific musculoskeletal pain. Mayo Clin Proc. 2003 Dec;78(12):1463-70.

18. Vitamin D Status and Bone and Connective Tissue Turnover in Brown Bears (Ursus arctos) during Hibernation and the Active State Peter Vestergaard.

19. Latitude studies on vitamin D and disease 2012, Autoimmunity Research Foundation

20. See #16.

22.
Testimonials

Here is an email I got 10/2012 from a lady who had chronic wound healing problems that seem to have been cured by high dose D3!

From: Janell

I am a 69 yo female who has suffered for the past 12 to 14 years with a bad back, overweight, etc. Since 2006, I have had Lap Band surgery (2006), Spinal fusion of L 2-3 and rebuild of L 1 and spending 34 days in a rehab facility (2008), removal of a mesh bladder sling 2010, rebuild of a bladder sling of my own tissues (Jan. 2011). The bladder sling rebuild resulted in an infection

which led into a wound that would not heal. In October of 2011, it was recommended that I go to a Wound Healing Clinic where I met with the staff and the doctor on a weekly basis to have the wound scraped out and the 'Wound Vac" replaced for another week. This continued through May, 2012 when I was told that, because the wound was not healing, I should return to my original surgeon, which I promptly did. He recommended a plastic and reconstructive surgeon to see if he could, perhaps, repair the wound so that it would heal.

In June of this year I bought myself a Kindle, and one of the first books I bought was yours, "Against Doctor's Orders!!"

This has literally been a life saver, and I can't thank you enough.

But, my saga continues. I now take 75,000 IU D3 daily along with 7 mcg of K2 daily. Is this enough K2?

At this time, 10/22/2012, I am feeling better than I have for years. Most of my back pain is gone and I can stand for a couple of hours with very little irritation pain. A knee injury from 8 or 9 years ago ha healed and my kneecap is back where it belongs. My left leg is continuing to heal from being semi paralyzed with no feeling from my hip to my toes. Though I will say that a Naproxen is necessary when the nerves reconnect and I get a 'shocking feeling'

I did have the surgery to make the wound start healing on July 26, 2012. It was a total success. I had two drains after surgery. One came out after two weeks and is completely healed. The one on the left side came out after 7 weeks, and only requires a Band-Aid to cover the drain area to prevent irritation from my underwear.

I am sending my new primary care doctor your name and e-mail. She believes that I am taking too much D3 and calcium. My levels on October 2 were D3 80 and calcium 112. This was when I started taking more K2. She is a new Doctor and is just learning. The med reports said I should be between 30 and 50 for my D3 levels, and I was only slightly high on the calcium levels. I have told her that I heavily participate in my own health care, so we shall see.

Again, thank you for sharing your knowledge. I feel human for the first time in years, and plan to continue for many years to come.

Oh, and I am losing weight again. Please feel free to contact me if you wish.

Janell

My Response-

WOW Janell

I am so happy for you..that really makes my month!..I get a lot of cure stories but yours sounds particularly amazing....

I renamed the book and it has been updated many times and has a lot more new information in it...

You ought to get a new copy upload it and read the new stuff there is lots of it..

Anyway....it is important to take the K2 ...what does K2 do? It activates the hormone osteocalcin..this hormone grabs calcium out of your blood and soft tissues and puts it in your bones when there is no K2 the osteocalcin goes in reverse and takes the calcium out of your bones and puts it into your blood and soft tissues....

So you want to take LOTS of K2 with your D3   you see D3 is dissolving and remodeling everything and if you use up your K2 the calcium can get into your blood and soft tissues...and cause problems.......this is why doctors are scared of it.....because they don't know about K2.....

I took 1 super K from www.lef.org   for every 10,000 iu of d3 a day.....so when I took 100,000 iu I was taking 10 super k's..their super Ks each have 1000 mcg of K1 also 1000mcg K2 of the mk4 type and 100mcg of the mk7 type (by the way 1000mcg = 1mg)

Mk4 comes from animals and is not as strong   Mk7 comes from bacteria and is much stronger....

now be careful.....some people have taken too much K2 and they complain of heart racing headaches and high blood pressure...

I just figured out that these are the symptoms of not enough calcium in your blood and heart..(hypocalcemia) ....so you have to thread the needle.....I would keep taking more and more until you finally get heart racing then back off a bit if you want to get tot the right amount to actually remove calcium from your soft tissues.......

anyway most people have no problems with the K2 levels I take...and www.lef.org even tells you to take twice as much K2 that I do...

so at 75,000 IU a day of d3   I would take 8 super K's or more to avoid any calcification risk...

oh and I would tell your doctor she should study up on d3 real quick and that you should be okay getting your blood level up to 90 minimum....maybe even 125 for awhile....the only risk of going to 100 to 200 is a slight increase in the risk of afib for those over 65 ....from the 5% normal risk to 12.5% for those with over 100 d3 levels....

however I am guessing K2 ameliorates this risk...read the review by Millard Ferguson and you see two surgeries did not cure his afib but high dose d3 and k2 did..and he is 91 hey thanks for writing , enjoy the updated book and please go to the Amazon website for the book and write a review and put all this information in it so others can know about it!!!

and please keep me posted I have you in the database!!!

all the best Jeff

A review from a British lady who had Crohn's disease, arthritis and depression for 50 years

5.0 out of 5 stars **All Doctors should be made to read this invaluable book. - ALSO SEE ADDITION 7 MONTHS LATER** 23 Jun 2013
By maggie
Format:Kindle Edition|
This book has helped me more than any health book I have ever read. For the last year I have had unbearable Arthritic pains resulting in swollen hands,fingers and wrists and pains in every joint and muscle. I could not sleep but was tired out all the time. I also have Crohn's disease which I have managed with a diet for over 50 years. Two weeks ago a friend sent me an article on this book. It made sense. I had a blood test and it came back as being Adequate. I live in UK. Measurements are different in US. I thought that perhaps I didn't need extra Vit D. I emailed Jeff who is extremely approachable and helpful and it appears that on the US scale my vitamin D levels were below even the reference range!! This is really criminal.

Immediately I started taking 4000 iu Vit D and also Vitk2. After 4 days I felt much better. On day 5 I took 12000iu and the pain dramatically decreased. I upped the dose to 16000 and again the same. I am now on 20000 and I have never felt so well and have only been taking it for just over a week. My energy is slowly increasing and I am now looking forward. I will write another review when I am further down the line to see if it helps with Crohns. I feel the research of this man has saved me.

7 MONTHS DOWN THE LINE

I have now been on Vit D3 & K2 for the last 7 months. My severe Arthritis has disappeared and my Crohns disease is being cured. I had not eaten bread for years and years so I decided to try some. I have been eating it for a month with no ill effects. If I did this before Vit.D I had debilitating pain. The depression I suffered from for years has gone. This is a big thing for me. I feel fantastic. In fact I feel better than I have done in my whole life. I only wish I had had Jeff Bowles book years ago.

A recent review from someone with Lupus

5.0 out of 5 stars Great Information!!, September 12, 2013

By T. Thielen (Albuquerque NM) - See all my reviews
(REAL NAME)

I am very fortunate to have found this ebook. I had a Vit D test on July 25, 2013 and my test number was 18. It did not surprise me because I have been at these low numbers for years and did nothing about it. My doctors were never concerned about it and neither was I since I did not know better. I am female and 54 years old. In 1997 my body started falling apart and fifteen doctors and thousand of dollars spent trying to find a solution to my medical problems. I was referred to different doctors for different problems. I have discoid lupus on my scalp which caused quite a bit of hair loss, horrible skin breakouts and lesions on my scalp, face, chest and arms. I started loosing my eyegrows and eyelashes. Talk about severe stress. I was at stage 5 adrenal fatigue, take thyroid medication and of course medication for the lupus problems. I could not heal with the different medications I took or the healthy foods I ate. I became allergic to the sun. If I did go outside I would break out in welts on my exposed skin. I found the e book and started taking 10,000 of Vitamin D3 with the K2 the following Monday. Four weeks later I had another blood test and my Vitamin D level was at 58. I am now seven weeks taking my Vitamin D3. My eyelashes, eyebrows and hair have started growing back in. I still have a way to go growing my scalp hair back in though. All of my welts have healed!! Nothing I did before would heal my skin. My skin is now very supple, it feels as if I have tons of lotion on. I had a root canal done two weeks ago and was put on penicillin for 10 days (endodontist said I had this problem for over a year) and for 5 of those days I stopped the Vitamin D3. My entire body started hurting again. I felt so bad. I immediately started my vitamins again and I was back to my old self again the next day. I am now able to spend time out in the sun again. It feels so good. Last week I spend time weeding my garden and got bit by several mosquitos. Usually these bites are very uncomfortable and I scratch my skin until it bleeds. NOT this time. I was bit and I did not feel any discomfort whatsoever. My skin never swelled from the bites nor did they itch. For me that was amazing. I have a doctors appointment soon and I will ask for a thyroid test and d level test to see where I am at. I want to get off of my medications. I have been wanting to up my Vitamin D3 to 20-30,000 UI. I still have a way to go. I have a bone spur and some other medical issues I want healed. The vitamins I now take are Andrews Lessmans Vitamin D3-2000UI (10,000) K1/K2 (1000), Calcium(2500) Magnesium (1200) per day. Again, thanks for the valuable information provided to us. I am planning to put my husband and brother on this program. They both need it! **My present doctor is learning as much as he can from me. I am his only patient that he knows of taking this much Vitamin D and he has noticed the huge improvement

A review from Dr. Donn Carroll

58 of 62 people found the following review helpful

5.0 out of 5 stars Cured My Incurable Psoriasis with 50,000/day in 2 months!! June 12, 2012

By Don Carroll

This is the most helpful book of the century. Jeff is a genius out of the box thinker to come up with an epic tome like this. He researches thousands of studies on D3 to find out the great benefits with almost zero side effects. Then he uses himself as an experiment to find the right dosage. The studies show almost every disease is eliminated with large dose D3 because it is a hormone naturally made in the body from the sun.
I just got back my lab results from using 50,000 units of D-3 with Vitamin K-2 MenaQ7 (Metabolic Maintenance) daily for 2 months. My test showed 150 ng/mL, this is in the high range of what most authorities say it should be but I hate to reduce it. Just four months ago I had the worst Psoriasis you could imagine covering my body. I could only sleep on my stomach I felt like Job from the Bible. My research found almost nothing that would help it. I started on a mostly raw vegan, gluten free diet with super foods and super herbs and no sugar and some cultured vegetables. I then began to take the D-3. I now feel so good and have had so many good results besides the disappearance of the Psoriasis. I

sleep like a baby my ganglion cysts are disappearing, my previously injured thumb is remodeling, my skin is not as dry, my prostate healed, restless leg gone and I could go on and on. I feel totally on top of the world.

If you have an ailment especially an incurable read this book. By the way I am taking Russell James TheRawChefAcademy.com internet course for the best raw food without sugar you could imagine.

A review from a man with afib

5.0 out of 5 stars This book will become a classic for vitamin D proponents April 26, 2012

By Millard Ferguson

I read this book

with interest because I have been taking large doses of vitamin D for more than 5 years. I should mention that I am a 91.5 year old male who started taking 5000 iu's of vitamin D 5 years ago, with 25(OH) D3 level of about 45 ng/ml.

I gradually increased my D intake and have been taking 12000 iu, with a 25(OH)D3 level of 90 to 97 for the past 2 years, along with vitamin K2. My blood work has not shown any significant changes over this period. Several things have occured in my health situation that now suspect, after reading Jeff's ebook, have been caused by my relatively high D level:

1. My atrial fibrillation (afib) has been cured, at least for the last 8 months, after the third cardioversion procedure, when my D3 level

was near 100 ng/ml.
The previous two attempts,unsuccessful, where done when my D
level was low.
2. After serving underhanded for the last 3 years, because of a
shoulder problem, I can now serve a tennis ball normally with no
pain.

Millard Ferguson

A review from a lady with severe COPD

To: jeffbo <jeffbo at aol dot com.
Sent: Fri, Mar 21, 2014 11:33 pm
Subject: Vit D Review

Hi Jeff, a few weeks back you had asked me to leave a review of
my experience so far with Vit D. I was not sure where to leave it
so I will write it here and give my permission to post it where ever
you feel it would be helpful to others.

I have been using High Dose Vit D for 11 weeks to date. I began
with 20 IU and gradually moved up to 80K IU by week 8. I began
using Vit D for the treatment of COPD. I am 44 and have been
battling symptoms for 11 years. I have never smoked or been
exposed to lung contaminants that I know of. I have tried many
Natural Treatments including other high dose herbs and many
Natural Modalities. All have been helpful for a time and in a
limited capacity. At the time of beginning Vit D, my symptoms
had become unmanageable and life threatening, increasingly by the
day. I had seemingly run out of options. So trying this so called
"Extreme" felt like a last ditch effort.

By week six I had noticeable improvement in breathing and
congestion and asthma. I would say a 40 -50% improvement.
However an unexpected improvement was that I no longer had
stomach pain in caused by eating grain. I discovered this by
accidentally consuming grain and had no pain. I then experimented

to see if it was just a fluke and NO it wasn't. I still don't consume grain intentionally, but I can if I want to.

I went through a period of 10 days of severe pain in my hip and back. I was aware It could be an effect of the Vit D healing these areas that had been painful for years. I did not back off of the D. After 10 days I was completely pain free in these joints. I also went through weeks of needing to sleep long hours. I knew I was healing so I just went with it. That lifted at week 10.

At week 8 I had a 75 percent improvement in Congestion, shortness of breath, asthma and coughing. And by week 10 I had NO symptoms of COPD!!!!

I have in week 11 I backslid some. I have continued on with the 80 IU Vit D and Vit K, but have had some MILD symptoms return. I have also experienced some irritability and depression that is uncharacteristic for me.

I plan to continue for at least six months while monitoring blood levels.

Thanks for all of the info you provided. I am grateful for the knowledge and for my results.

Sincerely Liz L*******

From someone with MS

5 of 6 people found the following review helpful

5.0 out of 5 stars Walking Again, April 27, 2013

By merola - See all my reviews

I have MS and hadn't walked in 3 years. AFTER mega dose of D I am now walking 30 feet with a walker.

From a guy with Plantar Fasciitis

7 of 9 people found the following review helpful

5.0 out of 5 stars I AM AMAZED! I HAVE HAD PLANTAR FASCIITIS FOR 2 YEARS AND 25,000/DAY CURED ME IN 2 WEEKS!!, July 15, 2012

By Fabian Laszlo - See all my reviews

I read this book trying to find something to help my mother's cancer. And it sounded so good I decided to try it myself.
I have been limping for 2 years with painful plantar Fasciitis in my foot. After 2 weeks of taking 25,000 a day
it is 100% gone....I am so happy.
Also a friend of mine with shoulder arthritis has been taking it for two weeks too and his pain is almost gone.
I live in brazil and cannot get Vitamin K2 so I am buying the Japanese food Natto form the Japanese restaurants down here
it is supercharged with Vitamin K2. Natto have 1103.4 mcg/100g.

From a guy with who knows what??

9 of 12 people found the following review helpful

5.0 out of 5 stars A million stars out of 5!!!, March 16, 2013

6 days ago I was dying, I'm not even kidding. For the last 18 years I've been suffering deeply. I'm 25. I spent 30 days in 6 different emergency rooms in 2012-2013, I saw 35 free Canadian Doctors that all couldn't help me (yes, thirty five). I had lost 75% of my muscle strength, 30% of my muscle coordination, 98 to 99% of my muscle endurance (yes, I couldn't even work 6 days ago), I was trembling all the time, couldn't bend over, couldn't do a push-up, massive depression, would go blind often during hypoglycemia, had extreme hypoglycemia, insulin resistance, skin vitiligo on my penis, very painful problem spots aches that made me hurt badly: a piece of broken bone inside my foot that felt like I was stepping on a small rock when I would walk, an ache I had in my back, a terrible ache in my wrist that I got from punching a door open 10 years ago, a terrible pain under my right foot I got from landing too hard 10+ years ago, a terrible jaw pain that never went away after having a wisdom tooth removed 7 years ago. Also, I've been having difficulty hearing (embarrassing to always ask people to repeat), I've been hungry my whole life, eating non-stop all the time, 4 to 10 meals per day.

First day I decided to do 50 000IU, the next day I did 150 000IU and 150 000IU on third day. 4th day 400 000IU, 5th day 714 000IU (Crazy dose), 6th day 200 000IU. Suddenly, all the problem areas on my body are healing, suddenly, the piece of bone in my foot dissolves overnight, I wake up all red, everything is healing, all aches are burning, my ears burn and then I sleep more, I realize I can hear twice as good, my blood sugar is now perfectly stable (no need for glucose meter anymore), I feel energized, no depression, the hypoglycemia being gone is so amazing I'd have given ALL my money to cure this horrendous disease, I'm not going blind anymore, my libido is through the roof, skin vitiligo starting to heal (base of grey hairs on my head are turning brown, base of pubic hair turning black again). Also, let me say that vitamin D3 isn't the only thing that did this, I also took vitamin K2, calcium and magnesium all together at huge doses for each of them. This is more than a miracle, this is enough for me to sue Doctors for keeping this secret away from me. Vitamin D3 is the greatest supplement I've ever done. I got my D3 at Costco in Canada: 2 bottles of 360 pills @ 1000IU for 6.82$ + sales taxes,

Also, the muscle weakness is nearly all gone. Muscle coordination is up by a lot. My muscle trembling is still present but going away fast, jeez, this is only day 6!

An email about pimples libido and other things

Dear Jeff,

Update on D3

I have been taking 2 capsules of 10,000 per day (3 weeks) and I tell you I now feel younger and my body is full of life. My Libido is fantastic for someone 75.

My wife started 2 weeks ago. She has some sort of skin itching problem on the legs, looks like "Psoriasis" she has this problem for about 14 months. Her doctor has prescribed many tablets and lotions and the problem persisted. Now after taking D3 the skin looks almost normal and the itching was gone within days of taking D3.

I gave some D3 capsules (10,000) for a friend to try, he ordered some and he has been taking them for about 2 weeks.

10 days ago he came to see me with his 15 yr old son whose face is full of pimples. I gave him a capsule immediately and told him to take 2 a day.

This morning his father came to see me and he told me his sons pimples have all but disappeared. My friend has a beautiful color in his face and he told me that he has never felt better. He does weight lifting and he says that when he did that he had muscle aches for 24 hrs now he says he lifts same weights and no aches. Hi Libido is high (he compares it to viagra)

Now Jeff I will fill you in on "Melatonin" powder.

I used to wake up at least 5 – 8 times per night to urinate. I never slept good.

I have been taking about Melatonin 1/6 teaspoon every night.

I only urinate 1 am and 6 am almost like clockwork. I have a very fulfilling sleep. I don't know about my hair yet.

Kind regards,

Sammy

A review from a lady with asthma and skin conditions

24 of 27 people found the following review helpful

5.0 out of 5 stars Pain disappearing & Asthma Improvement, April 7, 2012

By alaskadancingbear - See all my reviews

I began my search to reduce pain and improve my overall health when I came across this book. I read it entirely in one evening and placed an order the following day for the supplements. It has been years since I have been able to lie flat on my back at night without any discomfort. Within a week, I found myself sleeping on my back. The throbbing pain in my leg going from my ankle to my hip was keeping me awake and during the day it would center around my knee. When I reached 20,000IU of D3, it went away. I dropped to 10,000 and it returned. I'm back on 20,000 and pain free. A skin condition is showing improvement also. It's been a less than 3 weeks that I began documenting results and I am truly amazed. And, if you want to contact the author, read his book, he gives you his email address and he actually cares enough to respond... I wanted to update my review by noting the improvement in my chronic asthma. I was born full term but spent three days in an incubator because of my lungs. All my life I have struggled with the condition - even though I was a runner, I was always trying to catch my breath after the event. The virus that I recently caught would have put me in respiratory distress and the end result would have been pneumonia. I haven't had any difficulty breathing with the virus, only coughing. It's been a week now and today I'm almost completely back to better health and still taking the D3. I believe the D3 has had a significant role in my improved lung capacity. I'm barely using my rescue inhaler and I've cut down on my daily medications..I'm beginning the 30,000 dosage today...will see what this brings over the next two weeks and I'll update this review....Here's to better health for all...

Review by someone with dark circles under eyes

5.0 out of 5 stars Wow - Awesome Information on Vitamin D3 and Vitamin K, April 20, 2012

By Joann E. Rogers (Hutto, TX United States)

I don't know what to say, ordered the kindle ebook, read it shared it followed it. Within 3 days the dark circles under my eyes that were supposed to be from allergies were GONE! I have had aches and pains since a work accident when I was 32 and like the author I am in my early 50's and really tired of hurting all the time. So I am taking around 20,000 IU's a day right now the sublingual type with Vit K also. My neck and back feel a lot better and my fatigue is starting to lighten up. Only on it for a week and already seeing changes. THANK YOU for the information at such an affordable price!

From someone with depression

5.0 out of 5 stars Great results from following the authors advice, December 14, 2012

By otter30 - See all my reviews

I was intrigued by the title but skeptical of the claims. However the reasonable price swayed me.

The book is written in the spirit of "The 4 Hour Body". The author has come up with a very intriguing theory on how large doses of D3 could benefit us, and conducts an experiment on himself to verify aspects of the theory. He claims that he benefited greatly.

Well, I took his advice and am now up to 35000 IU a day after 4 months. I can wholeheartedly say that the authors advice has greatly benefited me. In addition to the resolution of general tiredness and overall joint pain/creakiness issues, an unexpected benefit was that I no longer take Prozac after being on it for over 18 years. I actually feel much better on the high D3 dose than I ever did from Prozac. Prozac prevents depression, the D3 actually makes you feel good.

Despite the book being a bit disjointed, I have to give it 5 stars because of the good that comes from following the authors advice. At this price, he is really doing a wonderful thing here.

Review by someone with many health problems

13 of 14 people found the following review helpful

5.0 out of 5 stars My own experiment, results, August 14, 2012

By kmisty19898 - See all my reviews

I am my third week of my experiment, and thought you might like to know the results I have so far. Just so you know I started with 30,000 IU daily of D3 with 200mcg K2. But I must admit (here's fodder for another book) I am also taking cayenne pepper twice daily. I use 1/4 teaspoon in 1ounce apple cider vinegar in 4 ounces of the hottest water I can stand. The hot water helps it absorb. But you can only use Heinz in the glass jar or home-made vinegar because the other stuff is synthesized.

RESULTS:

1-Haven't felt like this in 15 years at least! Even my friends are remarking that I seem "Perky" to them.
2-I am feeling some heavy pain in my very arthritic knee, and was thinking of cutting back, but I want the joint to "remodel".
3-I have been diagnosed with depression and schizo-effective disorder and see #1
4-The cracking of my knuckles is minimizing already.
5-I have degenerative disk disease and extruded disks in my back with arthritis. Something IS going on there I can feel it.
6-I use an exercise machine and have noticed that I have a much faster recovery time between sets than before, because I feel so good.
7-My eyes are being effected too, my night vision is getting better already and my vision seems sharper.
8-I am losing my appetite! And have lost a tad bit of weight!
9-I am very tired at the end of the day and have been sleeping through the night. I've had sleep disturbances for years and tried many different meds to no avail!

This is just what I have noticed thus far and it's just the beginning of the third week! I praise God that I found your book! I've been telling my friends with mixed reviews, but one couple have purchased the D3and K2 and I "gifted" them the book so they don't go astray somewhere and quit. I am on disability and don't receive much money but next month I plan to buy your "Alzheimer's" book. Thank you for pulling me back from the brink!

Review by someone with skin disease called PRP

5.0 out of 5 stars WOW. A cure for my skin disease (possibly), November 16, 2012

By Jaime Vendera ""Phoenix Earth" produc... (Ohio) (VINE VOICE)

WOW, this author should be a scientist!!! I cannot believe the lengths he went on his own to study D3. He should be paid by the government!

I accidentally stumbled across this book when browsing Kindle, and honestly, I'd usually skip over a book with such a long title on a plain yellow background, but something told me to stop and take a look. I'm so glad I did! I'm a lifelong sufferer of a skin disease called PRP (pityriasis rubra pilaris) and I have suffered severely for the last five years, with dry, inflamed skin, energy loss, blurred vision, low libido, etc., much worse than I have during my 30+ years of this affliction. Fed up with dermatological treatment, I started looking for natural alternatives.

When I found this book, vitamin therapy, or D3 for the matter, wasn't even a consideration. But I followed my gut and forked out $2.99. Off the but, I can tell you that this book reads like you are talking to the author, who is shooting words out of his mouth at 150 mph. i'm not saying that is a bad thing, I'm jut noting that he jumps from point to point, deeply explaining every little detail. But, if he didn't, I would not known the benefits and supposed dangers of D3. For one, I had no idea that D3 wasn't really a vitamin but a secosteroid. Well, that was a home run for me, because I've used a lot of Prednisone over the years to calm my inflamed skin, but that is some bad mojo for the body in the long run.

So, I ended up buying D3 and K2 as he suggested and started a daily regimen of 30,000 IU. It is already making differences in my body and it's only been a week! Patches of my skin are returning to normal, my energy levels are climbing again, (I'm back to cardio finally, no more looooong afternoon naps and my libido in increasing (honey, here I come, ha-ha.)

So, all in all I am sooooo thankful for this book. Though it is a long, read, it is very informative, as well, has some insights into diabetes that I think the doctors may want to stop and read. If only more minds were this inquisitive, we may solve world hunger, ha-ha. So, if you don't mind, I shall finally part from this review and purchase a few more of this author's books as I continue taking my D3 and reaping the benefits!

Sue's recent email:

I was tested & found deficient so started taking 2000 iu for 60 days, my knees that my doctor & orthopedic surgeon both told me needed replaced are so much better but still sore after standing a long time, so I increased to 10000 iu 2 weeks ago and knees are fine, also improved my fingers which had limited movement since I broke them 2 -3 years ago. Feel like a new person, get tested in another week to see what level is now. I can't believe such a simple fix!

I just had my eye appointment after taking D3 now for about 90 days, My eyesight had improved! It's official, my right eye went from +2.25 to +0.75 and left eye from +0.75 to -0.25. My near vision (reading) went from +2.75 to +2.50. Dr didn't believe it was from D3 but that's the only difference from last year. Same meds, same weight, etc. Assistants at both eye doctor's office and eyeglass place asked if I had had corrective surgery. Knees are also still improving, but can walk up & down steps now and able to stand longer without pain. Thank you Jeff Bowles for your book. I had no idea!

I have my regular doctor appointment next Monday with results of 2nd D3 level test and checkup. Boy is my doctor going to hear about it!!! What a surprise for him.
Thanks again for your book.
Suse

Mark's email re: actinic kertosis:

If I could play golf pain free again, I would be happy with that. Possibly some of these dreams can be realized through consistent D3 therapy.

Oh, and I took it to heart to go ahead and do k-2 therapy along with d-3 to avoid the wrong effect on the bones. I am taking greater than 80,000 ius d-3 daily. How much k-2 do you think I need to take with that? I weigh about 155 lbs.

Last March 2012 I fractured my spine falling off a ladder trimming a tree. My compression fracture fused just fine with lots of supplementation but it has been a struggle to regain strength in the ligaments. I also banged up my left knee pretty good but comparatively speaking a much lesser problem. I have pain in the knee and it is slightly swollen but my mobility is still there. In fact I have been sprinting 100 yard dashes as part of my exercise program. I have not had the knee scoped but i suspect a possible bone chip in the tissues cause it hurts when I kneel down on it or sit with it bent in my easy chair for very long. I am wondering if d-3 will rehab this knee.

I don't know if I mentioned it in my last email but the high d-3 has resolved my actinic keratosis. This is one of those irritating syndromes that doesn't allow you to be exposed out in the sun. You get a raised red rash on neck, forearms and legs. The sun makes the little red bumps itch and fester almost like poison ivy or something. I am a red headed fair skinned individual. This summer I was able to go outside and enjoy the sun (without sunscreen) for fairly lengthy durations, say 1-1/2 to 2 hrs without burning and without any effect on the rash bumps. Vitamin D is itself protective against UVA. Today the rash bumps are few in number.

A recent testimonial from someone who cured their lifelong bone spurs..& lost 30 pounds w/o trying:

This is one of the greatest books I have read in years.
I am an avid health reader and much similar to Jeff I do my own health experiments.

Here are a couple of observations of my own:
1: Per my podiatrist I had two of the largest bone spurs he had ever seen on my ankle. I got them when I was 16(I am 40 now) when I jumped off of the roof and landed on a bent foot. I did not break a

bone but the trauma took a few month's to heal and left me with two nasty spurs that would stay with me for the next 24 years. I put myself on 26000 iu of vitamin d3 for 9 months and both these spurs have disappeared completely. Really unbelievable.

2: I also lost 30 pounds without even trying (230 lb to 200 lb).

3: Also I used to get the cold/flu every year, this year it seems to have taken a vacation.

I have initiated a bunch of other health experiments using so called large dose vitamin D and I would update my review when I get an update.

A recent review: D3 and autism, thyroid medication, ganglion cysts, asthma:

5.0 out of 5 stars **Vitamin d3 has made wonders in our family. We are living proof of this** <u>Aledav</u>

Though the author writes like he is talking 100 miles per minute, it is very easy to follow right along with him. I think everyone should read this book. It's amazing how many people know nothing about vitamin d3 and are ready to criticize the information. A couple of years ago I went to a regular doctor visit and was asked the general questions about what supplements and medications I was currently taking. The doctor freaked out when I said I was taking 3000 iu daily and ordered a toxicity test for d3, which came back normal. I am currently taking 6000 iu daily and a ganglian cyst which I had for years has disappeared. I also went to my endocrinologist and my thyroid medication has been lowered for the first time ever and it has always been increased instead. I also have a 5 yr old son on the autism spectrum whom I've been giving 1200 iu daily. They just tested his d3 and it was low. The doctor told to increase it to 4000 iu daily. We have seen improvement in his speech, WAY BETTER EYE contact, and more social. He will get retested in December to see if we should increase it again. I am more than excited with the results we are experiencing. My daughter takes 3000 iu daily, and when she is off of it, her asthma bothers her. My husband takes 5000 iu and is thinking going up to 10000 iu. At our home, we have not had a cold or the sneefles in years (before taking d3 in these doses). Before people start talking negative, they should do some research and try it for them selves. Love the book and the information.

A recent review: D3 ganglion cysts, blood sugar , and appetite:

5.0 out of 5 stars **Enthusiasm to push me to do more researchM. R. "me"** (Chicago, IL United States)

While not a masterpiece of editing and style, this book is enthusiastic and has lots of research that you can go to yourself to get additional information. I have done a lot of Vitamin D research before, but this book inspired me to try to find information on large doses. This was also the first book that said anything about K2 - which is important to how Vit. D works. I do wish the author had been clearer about how long he took each mega-dose of D3, but each update the author does to the book seem to improve its flow incrementally. Read the book and catch some of the author's enthusiasm for D3.

I had been taking 10k IU of Vitamin D3 for over a year and had noticed improved moods. Then I got this book. I upped my D3 to 50k IUs a day on Oct. 1, 2013. I ordered K2 and started that along with it on about Oct.15th. About mid-month in October I realized that my ganglion cysts (which I have in both wrists) had retreated significantly. Now, on Nov. 1, I can't feel them at all. It is really hard to tell how long the author took each mega dose he talks about. That is why I think that getting your Vit. D levels tested will be very important. I just sent my test kit in and should have results soon. (I'll update this review when I get them.)

I have noticed that my blood sugar seems steadier - I don't crave carbs or get hungry as often. I think I may have taken my D3 too late on the day a few times and that has made it difficult to sleep, so now I try to take it early in the day. I have none of the aches and pains that friends the same age (mid-40s) complain about.

ETA: Got my results. Last year at this time, taking 10k IUs per day, I was at 66 ng/ml. Today, after 3 weeks at 50K IUs/day I am at (oops) 172 ng/ml. I may reduce my dose a bit, but I might not. I am taking my K2 and I feel great.

A recent review: Crohn's Disease Is Cured:

My Crohn's Disease Is Cured, Kurt W. Fuller

I must say that I literally stumbled onto this book. But the title rang true with me, so I bought it (Kindle version) for a very low price.

Around age 53, I was diagnosed with severe Crohn's disease. At the same time, I was diagnosed with prostate cancer. Though a number of different urologists were "foaming at the mouth" wanting to remove the prostate, I decided to try alternative medicine first (over the objections of everyone in knew).

Fortunately, I found a doctor (in a state halfway across the country) who practiced alternative medicine. He cured me of prostate cancer without surgery. However, he said that my Crohn's was far more dangerous to me in the long run. I said that I'd researched Crohn's thoroughly on the internet and that every site called the disease "incurable." He scoffed and said that my problem was a shortage of Vitamin D.

At the time, I was taking 1,000 IU of Vitamin D per day. The doctor recommended an increase to 2,000. When that didn't work, he changed the dose to 4,000. Then he went to 5,000. Then 10,000. Then 15,000. At 15,000 I finally began to see improvement. After 3-4 years, my symptoms disappeared.

I'm now 59. Oh how I wish I'd seen this book years ago. I can see now that the strategy was good, but the doses were way too small. I have friends with Crohn's who refuse to deviate from what "the doctor" says, despite their lack of success. Maybe if they read this book, they'd think differently. I couldn't recommend any book more strongly than this one.

A recent review: Cures acne in 1 month better than Acutane:

Jeff-Just wanted to give you an interesting update.
I have had my son on high dose D3 (and K2) for a month or so now. He is 19 and has had severe acne since about 16. He went on on Acutane when he was junior in high school and of course this dangerous drug worked; temporarily. I was reluctant to try this drug, however, it is hard enough being a teenager!
After about a year his acne returned.
I am happy to report that his face is almost completely cleared!

Cindy M.

A review from a lady trying to get pregnant for 3 years with in vitro fertilization:

Hello Mr. Bowles

I have been trying to conceive for 3 years with mild to moderate endometriosis. After three failed iui's, I knew something else was wrong like an autoimmune issue and decided to read a few books on my own. I came across your book on Amazon and bought a copy 2/26/13. I don't exactly remember what i started with but it was low, between 25-35. I started taking vit. D3 to get levels up high before another try, nothing to lose but give it a try. I bought 10,000 units, started at 50,000 units a day with the vit.k for about a month, then 30,000 a day for a couple weeks, and then 20,000 units a day until this blood test.

From: Advisory From: advisory@lifeextension.com
KADY@
Sent: Tuesday, March 19, 2013 3:08 PM
Subject: vitamin D

Your 25 hydroxy vitamin D blood level was 129 ng/ml. Stop your vitamin D for 2 weeks, after that resume at ½ the dose. Optimal range for 25 hydroxy D is 50-80 ng/ml. You can retest in about 2 months.

This was my level before I conceived in April 2013. I delivered a healthy baby in December 2013. Your book was a tremendous help.
Thank you so very much.
K.B

From a man with severe dandruff, IBS, lower back pain, & bleeding gums:

Hi Jeff,

Your book has changed my life.

Severe dandruff of 10 years gone.

IBS of 20 years 50% gone.

Lower back pain 2 years, 100% gone.

Bleeding gums gone.

Many thanks, and kind regards.

All the best.

Richard C.
South Africa

From a man with a 20 year staph infection:

Hi Jeff,

aftera long a time, I finally found what I have for 20 years, STAPHYLOCCOCCUS and RINGWORM.

let me know if K2 is beneficial in this case too. I was taking 25k d3 + 2caps K2 for almost 2 months and it was better with the eyes but dont know how it affects staph infection.

I will try again 50k D3 DAILY. so please let me know.

Hi Julian-great news

getting the right diagnosis is often 90% of the battle.....

I expect most infections should fall to D3 as the high doses super charge your immune system.......

you will be the first I have heard attacking staph with it...

thanks-Jeff

Hello Jeff

2 days 50000 IU VITAMIN D3+ k2 shows good results. i have staphyloccocus on head in the eyes, face, mouth etc.

Klin Wochenschr. 1977 May 15;55(10):507-8.

[Studies on the antimicrobial effect of vitamin D (author's transl)].

[Article in German]
Feindt E, Ströder J.

Abstract
In in vitro studies vitamin D3 proved inhibitory on strains of Staphylococcus aureus, Streptococcus pyogenes, Klebsiella pneumoniae. Escherichia coli, and Candida albicans. In the presence of $5 \times 10(4)$-$9 \times 10(4)$ IU/ml vitamin D3 the organisms were killed or reacted with a marked growth inhibition.

It is proved vitamin d3 is A MIRACLE. but I have to test it for at least 2 months but for now i found a very high RELIEF.

About the author

Jeff T. Bowles is no more qualified to write about these things than you are except for the fact that he has spent many weeks, months and years researching these things as his avid hobby. Please do not rely on any credentials he may or may not have but please just evaluate the words and ideas in the article and do your own research and critical thinking. There are many fools with PhDs. Relying on credentials to evaluate an argument is just a sad form of intellectual laziness.

CPSIA information can be obtained at www.ICGtesting.com
Printed in the USA
LVOW04s1628161214

419118LV00018B/900/P